From Enslavement to COVID-19

From Enslavement to COVID-19

A History of African American Health and Labor

Joe William Trotter Jr.

The University of North Carolina Press CHAPEL HILL

This book was published with the assistance of the Lilian R. Furst Fund of the University of North Carolina Press.

Set in Merope Basic by Westchester Publishing Services
Manufactured in the United States of America

Library of Congress Cataloging-in-Publication Data
Names: Trotter, Joe William, Jr., 1945– author
Title: From enslavement to COVID-19 : a history of African American health and labor / Joe William Trotter Jr.
Description: Chapel Hill : The University of North Carolina Press, [2025] | Includes bibliographical references and index.
Identifiers: LCCN 2025013864 | ISBN 9781469690841 cloth | ISBN 9781469690858 paperback | ISBN 9781469683348 epub | ISBN 9781469690865 pdf
Subjects: LCSH: African Americans—Health and hygiene—History | Medical care—United States—History | African Americans—Employment—History | Racism against Black people—United States—History | BISAC: SOCIAL SCIENCE / Ethnic Studies / American / African American & Black Studies | MEDICAL / Health Policy
Classification: LCC RA448.5.B53 T76 2025 | DDC 362.1089/96073—dc23/eng/20250606
LC record available at https://lccn.loc.gov/2025013864

Cover art: *Hospital Union Workers*, by Charles "Teenie" Harris. Getty Images.

For product safety concerns under the European Union's General Product Safety Regulation (EU GPSR), please contact gpsr@mare-nostrum.co.uk or write to the University of North Carolina Press and Mare Nostrum Group B.V., Mauritskade 21D, 1091 GC Amsterdam, The Netherlands.

This book is dedicated with love and appreciation
to health care providers among and beyond
my family members and friends:
Salena Harris Johnson
Dr. Marva Ann Jones
Marva Louise Bell Dodson
Dr. Tanya L. Trotter
Myna Jo Shegog
Dr. Alexis Grimes Trotter
Kersha Diebel Trotter
Otis Trotter

Contents

Illustrations

Acknowledgments

It is a pleasure to acknowledge some of the many people who helped make this book possible. First and foremost, I am indebted to William A. Darity Jr., Gwendolyn L. Wright, and Lucas Hubbard for an opportunity to contribute a chapter to their timely collection of essays, *The Pandemic Divide: How COVID Increased Inequality in America* (Duke University Press, 2022). Produced amid the ravages of the coronavirus pandemic, my essay, "Labor History and Pandemic Response: The Overlapping Experiences of Work, Housing, and Neighborhood Conditions," established the intellectual foundation for this book. However, for encouraging the transformation of this chapter into a full-length study, I thank my editor Neils Hooper of the University of California Press. As I completed the first draft of *Building the Black City: The Transformation of American Life* (University of California Press, 2024), Niels expressed interest in publishing a book that would address the escalating demands of the pandemic for deeper and more systematic historical perspectives on Black health and health care. *From Enslavement to COVID-19: African American Labor, Health, and History* is a product of that conversation.

A variety of other institutions, individuals, and events also fueled the production of this book. They include, to name a few, a Zoom lecture on the racial impact of the pandemic for the innovative undergraduate course "COVID-19: What History Can Teach Us," at Carnegie Mellon University (CMU); an in-person Howard Mahan Lecture on "African American Health, History, and COVID-19," at the University of South Alabama in Mobile; a virtual talk, "Reflections on Race, History, and COVID-19," at the Reid Temple AME Church, Glenn Dale, Maryland; and, most notably, a Zoom faculty research seminar on my plan for transforming the *Pandemic Divide* essay into a book. Thanks to Emanuela Grama, director of CMU's history department faculty research seminar, for organizing a well-attended, highly engaged, and helpful discussion of the book's conceptual framework, argument, and evidence. For enhancing the writing of this book, I am also indebted to the ongoing editorial work of Susan Whitlock.

I am also grateful to my colleagues Ezelle Sanford and Chante Boyd for an opportunity to present my work in their innovative undergraduate "Grand Challenge Course: You Make Me Sick." Ezelle also enhanced this study by generously sharing with me his extraordinary knowledge of the Black health care experience and historiography.

This book also benefited from the indispensable encouragement, comments, and suggestions of anonymous readers and staff for The University of North Carolina Press as well as longtime colleagues and friends. At the UNC Press, many thanks to Debbie Gershenowitz, executive editor, and acquisitions assistant Alexis Dumain for their enthusiastic response and support for this book. Among colleagues and friends, I am indebted most notably to Earl Lewis at the University of Michigan; Jacqueline Jones at the University of Texas-Austin; and Ronald Lewis at West Virginia University. As a work of historical synthesis, the scholarship of numerous colleagues constitutes the primary evidence for this study.

For supporting my work as Giant Eagle University Professor of History and Social Justice and Director of the Center for Africanamerican Urban Studies and the Economy (CAUSE), I am much obliged to the Giant Eagle Corporation and to Carnegie Mellon University, especially CMU President Farnam Jahanian, Provost Jim Garrett, Dean Richard Scheines, and department head Nico Slate. In addition, my CAUSE assistant and program coordinator Arlie Chipps provided able support services for all phases of this book, especially securing and gaining permission for use of copyrighted images. Reinforcing my work over the years, my colleagues Joel Tarr and Wendy Goldman in the history department have also been vital sources of support and friendship.

Above all, my family, the "Trotter-14" (now 12) and my late wife H. LaRue Trotter continue to inspire and make possible all that I do, including the writing and publication of this book. Finally, conceptualized and written in the throes of the global pandemic, this book is dedicated with deepest appreciation and gratitude to the health care professionals in my life and the life of the nation. Their dedication and sacrifices for the lives of others are immeasurable. These esteemed health professionals include, most notably, my great niece Dr. Alexis Grimes Trotter, a 2024 recipient of the PhD in environmental health from the University of Minnesota, my own PhD alma mater.

From Enslavement to COVID-19

Introduction

For a brief moment at the onset of the coronavirus (COVID-19) pandemic, disturbing reports circulated that African Americans "were not being severely affected" by the disease "or were less likely to be infected" than other populations. As the virus swept across the world, theories of Black people's immunity to COVID-19 "spread rapidly and widely" on social media. In an influential blog post on the subject, public health scholars and medical historians Chelsey Carter and Ezelle Sanford noted that such claims, coupled with misleading labels like "Kung Fu Flu" and the "China Virus," were not just "racist and xenophobic," but they were also "dangerous to *everyone's* health." Mounting evidence of alarming racial disparities quickly demolished the foundation of such erroneous early reports. The emerging racial profile of the pandemic underscored the need for deeper historical perspectives on the nation's public health crisis. Popular media and academic discussions soon started to acknowledge how the historic concentration of African Americans in dangerous and unhealthy work and living environments exposed them to disproportionately higher disease and death rates than their Euro-American counterparts.[1]

The recurring outbreak of epidemics and pandemics like COVID-19 compound and even confound ongoing racial disparities in the well-being of Black people. Understandably, recent discussions of health inequities in today's world often unfold with insufficient historical context for fully understanding the origins of both class and racial inequality in the diagnosis, treatment, and cure of disease. Unequal health and health care emerged among the first generation of African people on American soil. Such inequities were closely intertwined with the rise of white supremacist medical science, physician practices, and public health service policies as well as the debilitating work and living conditions of enslaved and later free people of color. Expanding bodies of medical research repeatedly underscore the close correlation between the "socioeconomic status" of Blacks and their mental and physical conditions at different moments in time. Lethal labor and living environments persisted and even intensified in the face of sometimes dramatic social transformations, including the forced migration of some 1.5 million African Americans from the Upper to the Lower South during

the early nineteenth century; the Great Migration and the rise of the industrial working class during the twentieth century; and the emergence of a predominantly low-wage service sector Black workforce in today's transnational
postindustrial economy.[2]

Closely intertwined with these changing moments in the nation's history,
African Americans (poor and working-class Black men and women as well as
the emerging Black medical profession) formed their own system of health
care. They challenged white supremacist medical science and sought to cure
themselves. But African Americans did not act entirely alone. The medical
rights movement forged significant, if tenuous, interracial networks of support with sympathetic white allies. Both the interracial and distinctively African American medical rights movements not only enhanced the health of
Black families and their communities but also reinforced the larger fight for
freedom and full citizenship rights across all categories of African American
life. Whatever their mode of organizing (class, cross-class, interracial, or
other), African Americans fought for their own livelihood and political
citizenship against the backdrop of racist ideas and practices in the healing
profession; ongoing but shifting forms of labor exploitation; and class and
racial limits on their access to livable housing, nutritious food, and medical
treatment.

Taken out of historical context, COVID-19-related conditions and deaths
among African Americans can be misinterpreted as anomalous. This brief
book, centered on four historical periods, argues that rather than being
anomalous, the fight for adequate health care and beneficial social service
policies parallel the movement of Blacks from slavery to freedom. Building
upon an expanding range of innovative studies on African American urban,
labor, social, and medical history since the transatlantic slave trade, this
study emphasizes how the labor requirements of work shaped the African
American encounter with disease. Further, it stresses how white medical
professionals and public health officials developed stereotypes about the susceptibility of Black people to disease and denied essential medical care to
the most vulnerable constituency of the country's total population, including the mentally ill.

Until the onset of the Civil War and the emancipation of enslaved people,
both popular and professional white opinion denied the existence of mental
illness among African Americans, mainly motivated by a desire to keep African Americans at work producing profits for economic, cultural, and political
white elites. In the case of the fugitive slave, however, contemporary slave
owners and their medical allies considered the widespread phenomenon of

running away (described as "drapetomania") as a "mental illness" rather than a quest for freedom from human bondage. According to physician Samuel A. Cartwright, drapetomania was "as much a disease of the mind as any other species of mental" disorder, but even that, he argued "was much more curable, as a general rule."[3]

In the rare instances where whites acknowledged mental illness among African Americans, they attributed such sickness to the stress of freedom rather than the products of enslavement and its impact on African Americans, even in cases where they managed to win their freedom. Most important, however, *From Enslavement to COVID-19* demonstrates how people of African descent, including poor and working-class Blacks, repeatedly built upon their own legacy of activism and community-building to improve their physical and mental conditions. They devised myriad programs and strategies designed to combat inequality and discrimination in the nation's health care system.

Chapter 1 explores the employment of enslaved African labor to cultivate diverse cash-producing staple crops, including tobacco, rice, sugar, and cotton. This chapter gives close attention to variations in the labor requirements of each crop, but accents the ways that enslaved labor from crop to crop took a huge emotional and physical toll on the lives of African people. Certain conditions, including long hours, severe corporal punishment, and inadequate medical treatment, diminished differences between crops and exposed Black people to high levels of sickness and death. This chapter also calls attention to the deleterious impact of white racist medical practices and ideas on Black people, including unethical and deadly medical experimentation on African American bodies. Under extraordinarily adverse circumstances, however, enslaved people did not rely solely on the planters' medicine. They created their own internal medical system. Drawing partly upon medical knowledge inherited from their West African culture and history, they worked mightily to heal themselves, both physically and spiritually. Over and over again, they challenged racist claims that "freedom" rather than the harsh conditions of enslavement and later disfranchisement of free people of color made them "crazy" as well as physically ill.[4]

In the wake of the Civil War and the emancipation of some 4 million people of African descent, the small family-based sharecropping system gradually supplanted the large plantation (with its overseer and gang labor) as the principal labor system employing newly emancipated people. Chapter 2 shows how postbellum Black people embarked upon a determined quest for landownership as the surest route to better health as well as full citizenship in the nation, but this dream faltered under a relentless upsurge of violent white resistance. Growing numbers of African Americans entered sharecropping agreements as another route to medical as well as political citizenship and economic democracy. This arrangement also quickly deteriorated into an oppressive system of labor exploitation, "perpetual debt," disfranchisement, violence, and high rates of sickness, disease, and death.

Following the Civil War and the general emancipation of Black people, professional psychiatry as well as popular white newspapers, magazines, and journals reiterated and intensified beliefs that the pressures of freedom and not human bondage and its afterlife accounted for increasing evidence of mental illness among African Americans. Psychiatry would acknowledge the growing incidence of mental disorder among emancipated people as a consequence of the Civil War. It would also open its doors to mentally ill African Americans on a segregated and unequal basis, partly as a way to secure much needed federal funds (including resources of the Freedmen's Bureau) to keep the profession and its mainly state-funded mental institutions alive.

Rather than expanding the scope of its earlier "moral therapy" for white inmates to include newly emancipated Blacks, professional psychiatry revamped treatment based on the exploitation of African American labor in the service of the institution itself. Still, African American postbellum farm laborers and sharecroppers built upon their vibrant antebellum tradition of medical activism and took a commanding role in the development of programs to improve their own health and living conditions. They registered these remarkable accomplishments against the larger backdrop of white supremacist medical science and practices that not only misinterpreted but also grossly neglected the medical needs (both physical and psychological) of Black people.[5]

By the late nineteenth century, rising numbers of sharecroppers abandoned the land for life and labor in the urban industrial sectors of the nation's rapidly expanding economy. This movement accelerated during the Great Migration of the twentieth century as an estimated 8 million African Americans departed the agricultural South for life and labor in workplaces and homes in the urban South, North, and West between World War I and 1970. Chapter 3 examines the rise of the Black urban industrial working class and its impact on the health of Black families and their communities. While migrants celebrated their movement into the urban industrial centers of the nation as a "New Jerusalem" and "Land of Hope," among other biblical terms, this chapter shows how they nonetheless labored on racially segregated and unequal terms in the most dangerous and unhealthy jobs in the industrial workforce, including most notably the steel industry, coal mines, the auto industry, and meatpacking establishments nationwide. Toxic work environments took a huge toll on the physical and spiritual well-being of industrial workers and dampened their "Land of Hope."[6]

As the twentieth century unfolded, the medical establishment also changed as a result of the new science of genetics. But the new science reinscribed older notions about the inherent biological and intellectual inferiority of Black people as the principal source of their disease and suffering. Certain ideas about the hereditary inferiority of Black people persisted into the new century and undermined African American access to adequate medical services for both physical and mental illness. Industrial-era Black Americans did not suffer quietly, however. Inspired by their history of medical justice struggles, they launched a plethora of grassroots movements to change the conditions under which they lived, worked, and received medical treatment during the industrial age. Their efforts also fueled the emergence of medical care alongside jobs and housing as key demands of the larger Black Freedom Movement.

In the years following World War II, the struggle for Black freedom undercut the American system of medical apartheid and opened the door for increasing numbers of African Americans, especially middle-class Blacks, to gain access to predominantly white medical institutions. The integration of African Americans into previously all-white hospitals and clinics precipitated the demise of the established Black medical infrastructure in some cities. These changes coincided with the rapid decline of the manufacturing economy; they also signaled the rise of a new class and racially divided postindustrial medical regime in rural, urban, and suburban America. Chapter 4 probes the transformation of African American work, housing, health, and living conditions as the industrial economy slipped away and the digital, postindustrial age took shape.[7]

The emergence of the digital age, which is still underway, has included multiple shifts in the health, lives, and livelihood of Black people and the nation. These momentous changes include, most notably, increasing use of new electronic medical recordkeeping practices; steady movement toward "personalized medicine" (focused on a fine-tuned understanding of a person's genetic makeup, diet, lifestyle, and environment) rather than a one-size-fits-all approach to the diagnosis, prevention, and treatment of disease; and, most importantly for this study, a fundamental shift in the types of work available for the vast majority of poor and working-class Black Americans.[8]

Rising numbers of working-class Blacks toiled in jobs without the benefit of union representation, retirement plans, and medical insurance packages. In the face of these new challenges to their health and well-being, the nation's African American community opened a new chapter in its long fight for medical justice and equal access to health care. By exploring the full scope of issues—the historical dimensions of labor, housing, and neighborhood conditions; racial interpretations and treatment of mental and physical illness; discriminatory public and private health care policies; and the African American struggle for full medical as well as economic and political citizenship—this book aims to reinforce and deepen public, academic, and policy discussions of race, labor, African Americans, and the COVID-19 pandemic. Above all, however, it is my hope that readers of this book will see more clearly how COVID-19 is part of a long history of Black medical struggles across North America and the transatlantic world—dating back to the advent of human bondage before the Civil War and the rise of the United States as a new republic.

CHAPTER ONE

Enslavement

Introduction

After surviving the horrors of the Middle Passage, a half million enslaved Africans disembarked in North America during the transatlantic slave trade. Slavery proved an exacting system, demanding much of the enslaved and taking much from them, beyond their labor. A racial ideology of alleged inferiority offered the intellectual underpinnings for slavery and the treatment of Black people. As a result, disease, injury, and death amounted to new hazards for those who survived the Middle Passage. This chapter traces that toll and the myriad ways African Americans tried to improve their health outcomes. It argues the fight for physical and mental well-being changed in lockstep with the crop grown, the racial propaganda produced, and the development of Black communities able to assert their places in a political economy predicated on their subordination.

Europeans quickly turned to enslaved African labor to produce a variety of staple crops for international markets, while de-emphasizing the degree to which slavery maimed, injured, and killed. The labor requirements of staple production varied from crop to crop, but the work regimen in sugar, rice, tobacco, and cotton took a huge toll on the health and lives of African people. While some diseases cut across all categories of work, living, and social conditions, others like chronic respiratory disorders were closely aligned with particular occupations.[1] Whatever diseases afflicted the bodies and minds of enslaved African Americans, however, Euro-American slaveholders and commercial elites downplayed the destructive physical and emotional impact of work, corporal punishment, and environmental conditions on the health of Black people.

On the one hand, following the logic and lead of the emerging medical profession, white supremacists embraced anti-Black conceptions of disease and sickness as products of African Americans' presumed inherent physiological and mental weaknesses as a race. On the other hand, they also invoked innate race-based factors to explain the apparent immunity of some Blacks to certain debilitating diseases like malaria and yellow fever. At the same time, both popular opinion and the emerging psychiatry profession rarely acknowledged the existence of mental illness among enslaved people. When they did, they downplayed its severity and accented the swift return of the mentally ill back to their regular work routines.

Such racially biased ideas and health practices reinforced the deadly impact of harsh labor and living conditions on enslaved people. They also set the stage for ongoing African American efforts to create their own system of health care to counter the effects of racist medical science. As such, they determined to diagnose, treat, and cure themselves. Their fight for good health and access to effective medical treatment was strengthened by the larger struggle to abolish human bondage. They aimed to gain full medical as well as political citizenship in the United States of America.[2]

White Supremacist Health Science and Healing Practices

The western medical profession, shaped by racial perceptions, gradually emerged during the late eighteenth and early nineteenth centuries. European and Euro-American physicians placed the acquisition of expert knowledge on Black bodies at the center of their aggressive campaign to establish medicine as a profession—replete with its own special modes of diagnosis, treatment, and cure of disease. As historical sociologist Paul Starr concludes in his massive synthesis of American medical history, western medical science laid claim to "an elaborate system of specialized knowledge, technical procedures, and rules of behavior" that governed medical ideas, education, and practices over the next century.[3]

"Medicalizing Blackness"

Based on skin pigmentation, the medical profession defined Blacks and whites as fundamentally different people, physiologically and intellectually, with different susceptibility and immunity to disease. Beginning with the eighteenth-century observations of Charleston, South Carolina's John Lining and Philadelphia's renowned abolitionist and physician Benjamin Rush, the notion of African Americans' innate immunity to yellow fever and malaria took strong hold in North America. Such beliefs not only ignored the impact of environmental and epidemiological conditions on African American health, but it also minimized and virtually erased the suffering of Black people who contracted these diseases. In 1826, Phillip Tidyman, a South Carolina physician and planter, declared in a Philadelphia journal of medicine that Blacks in the rice fields were unaffected by malaria, which he said was "so hostile to the white inhabitants." Tidyman then explained that affected Blacks required "little medicine to rid him of this insidious enemy."[4]

Of course, such observations were not without scientific explanation. By the twentieth century, research on sickle cell would show those who carried the disease or the trait had some immunities against malaria. But the disease could be otherwise debilitating and often terminal. Moreover, not all Africans doomed to work in Carolina rice fields had this genetic permutation. Black biological superiority in specific contexts lost out to the more pervasive sense that Blacks were biologically inferior to whites, which found its way into both general and scientific journals. Africans were presumably "innately" weaker people physically than whites and thus more prone to contracting a broader range of diseases than their Euro-American counterparts. Such biased ideas persisted over time and became "readily acceptable and widely circulated" within different temporal, geographic, and spatial contexts.[5] Early nineteenth-century medical theorists Richard L. North, John Shecut, and others carried these ideas forward. By the beginning of the Civil War, the so-called Big Three—physicians and medical scientists Georges Cuvier and George Lyell and British biologist and naturalist Charles Darwin—had emerged at the center of popular and professional opinion about race and medicine.[6]

White medical professionals were determined to sketch out regimens for various diseases on the assumption that Black and white bodies were different and required racially calibrated cures appropriate to their genetic makeup. Southern medical and popular journals offered regular and ongoing outlets for such ideas and health practices. In 1856, the planter and physician W. C. Daniell published an article in *DeBow's Review*, an agricultural journal, on a deadly case of "lockjaw" that had killed large numbers of Black babies on one Louisiana sugar plantation. According to Daniell, the infant deaths were caused by the ingestion of their mother's contaminated breast milk during roughly the first two weeks following birth. The article proposed a remedy, tailored specifically to treat Black rather than white women and their infants. The remedy entailed "feeding the newborn 'on sweet oil and molasses as to keep the bowels loose' and having 'the mother's breasts freely drawn and daily emptied of their milk . . . in any one of several ways; by the nurse, the midwife, another and older child, *or by a puppy* [my italics].'"[7]

Early Euro-American medical practitioners also devised racially biased definitions and cures for mental illness. In 1845, in its second edition, the *American Journal of Insanity* published a short essay titled "Exemption of the Cherokee Indians and Africans from Insanity." The article forcefully argued that it was white people's superior intellect and advanced civilization that exposed them to greater bouts of insanity than the simpler life of "primitive mental types" like the Africans and Native Americans. In other words, as literary critic and activist Mab Segrest notes, "white insanity equaled white mental superiority."[8] Author of the groundbreaking 2020 study *Administrations of Lunacy*, Segrest situates the roots of the professional conceptualization, treatment, and study of insanity in the racialized ideology, practices, and development of the Georgia State Lunatic, Idiot, and Epileptic Asylum, founded in 1842. Located in Milledgeville, the state's old capital city, this institution set the stage for the unequal treatment of mental illness along racial and class lines. Although this phenomenon had its beginnings in antebellum Georgia, it soon influenced racialized psychiatric ideas and practices across the United States.[9]

During the early nineteenth century, the historical records included significant accounts of mental illness among enslaved people. Such accounts described the incidence of Black mental disorders in similar language used to describe whites as "deranged," "slightly deranged," and "lunatic."[10] Despite such references to enslaved people in the plantation records, mental health professionals almost uniformly described Blacks as people with little incidence of mental illness. In their view, the childlike mental capacity and lifestyle of enslaved and free people of color alike inoculated them from the complexities of life experienced by independent, responsible, and free white adults. Over and over again, early professional psychiatry as well as lay white opinion dubbed people of color as a people with few cares.

On rare occasions when Black people exhibited symptoms of insanity, white mental health professionals considered such cases as ephemeral—presumably because Black people had an inner capacity to recover from such bouts quickly and resume their regular work regimen in the interests of their employers or owners. In 1846, in Petersburg, Virginia, one local practitioner, Dr. Joseph E. Cox, declared that after fifteen years of practice in the neighborhood, "I can call to mind no case of a slave that remained as a confirmed lunatic." Another Virginia practitioner, Dr. John Minson Galt II, superintendent of the Eastern Lunatic Asylum in Williamsburg, attributed the paucity of insane slaves to the hard work that enslavement entailed. According to Galt, bond labor strengthened the "constitution [of the enslaved] and enables it to resist physical agents, calculated to produce insanity."[11]

In testimony before the US Senate in 1848, even Dorothea Dix, the famous nineteenth-century crusader on behalf of the insane, reported that there were "comparatively few examples" of insanity among African Americans and Native Americans. Dix began her crusading work on behalf of the mentally ill in the Massachusetts prison system during the early 1840s, but she soon expanded her work across the state and nation, including the South. Because her work underscored the mistreatment of the mentally ill in states in the otherwise antislavery North, her efforts attracted sympathetic responses from the slaveholding Southern states. According to her biographer, Dix in effect "turned her back on the prejudice, hate, and violence of the slave system. . . . For her, the slave seems barely to have existed."[12]

By the late antebellum years, as the "asylum" for the "insane" spread across the nation, there was a growing convergence in Northern and Southern ideas about the diagnosis and treatment of mentally ill people of African descent. Across regional lines, African Americans occupied the cellar of the emerging mental health system. Responses to evidence of mental disorders among Blacks nonetheless varied somewhat from place to place within the North and South. In the South, African Americans were integrated with whites in Maryland, segregated in Kentucky, and excluded in Georgia, Mississippi, and Tennessee. Similarly, in the North, the Massachusetts General Hospital excluded Black patients, while both the Government Hospital for the Insane in Washington, DC, and the New York City Almshouse provided segregated quarters for Black inmates. But the treatment of the mentally ill was considered "deplorable" even among whites, and more so for African Americans. To take one example, a contemporary observer described the New York City facilities for African Americans as "a scene of neglect, and filth, and putrefaction, and vermin . . . a scene the recollection of which are too sickening to describe."[13]

Unethical and Deadly Experimentation

Emergence of the modern western medical profession exacerbated the health challenges confronting people of African descent. Enslaved and later free people of color were not only the subjects of racist thinking about disease and health care; they were also victims of neglect as well as unethical and deadly medical experimentation. No other ethnic or racial group suffered the widespread surgical removal of skin as did Blacks, with experiments done to satisfy the curiosity of white physicians bent on proving innate differences between Black and white people. In a careful study of the "voluminous literature of skin color" published in Europe between 1675 and 1810, historian Renato Mazzolini reported the dissection of some thirty-eight African bodies. Not only were white bodies apparently exempt from these incisions, but "not a single Amerindian or Asian was opened for this purpose."[14]

During the antebellum years, word spread globally about the "heroic surgical exploits" of American doctors based on the availability and use of enslaved Black bodies. Ready access to the enslaved bodies of Black people represented a sure way for aspiring white physicians to enhance their standing in the medical field. In 1857, Dr. John Butts, a Princeton, Mississippi, physician shipped the "freshly amputated arm" of a twenty-four-year-old female slave to the well-known New Orleans physician, educator, and journalist Dr. Erasmus Darwin Fenner. The woman's arm arrived at Fenner's office with a detailed case history report of the afflicted limb. According to historian Stephen C. Kenny, the surrender of the arm enabled a backwoods country doctor like Butts to cultivate ties to elite physicians like Fenner and his colleagues at the New Orleans School of Medicine. Butts's deed received extensive notice in the prestigious *New Orleans Medical News and Hospital Gazette*. His "specimen" also gained additional professional and public attention as part of an exhibit in one of the rising number of medical museums that spread across the antebellum South to help educate aspiring young doctors. African Americans provided the bulk of these popular exhibits of human body parts.[15]

The Alabama physician James Marion Sims provides the most notorious example of nineteenth-century medical experimentation on Black people. Sims performed vaginal surgeries on Black women in Montgomery, Alabama, between 1845 and 1852. Groundbreaking studies by Deirdre Cooper Owens, Harriet A. Washington, and others provide critical insights into this painful history of experimentation on Black bodies. Sims initially covered up his use of Black subjects at his hospital for the treatment of enslaved women suffering from "versico-vaginal fistulae, a common obstetrical condition that caused incontinence, and that was brought on by trauma and by the vaginal and anal tearing women suffered in childbirth."[16] As Washington put it, "Each surgical scene was a violent struggle between the slaves and physicians and each woman's body was a bloodied battleground." At the same time, paradoxically, as we will see, according to Cooper Owens, enslaved women attendants during these operations acquired and later imparted important knowledge that would help to lay the foundation for modern gynecology.[17]

Sims later moved to New York, where he continued to experiment on the bodies of African Americans as well as working-class Irish immigrant women. Enslaved men were also regular subjects of medical experimentation. In 1847, for example, the enslaved man John Brown escaped from the Clinton,

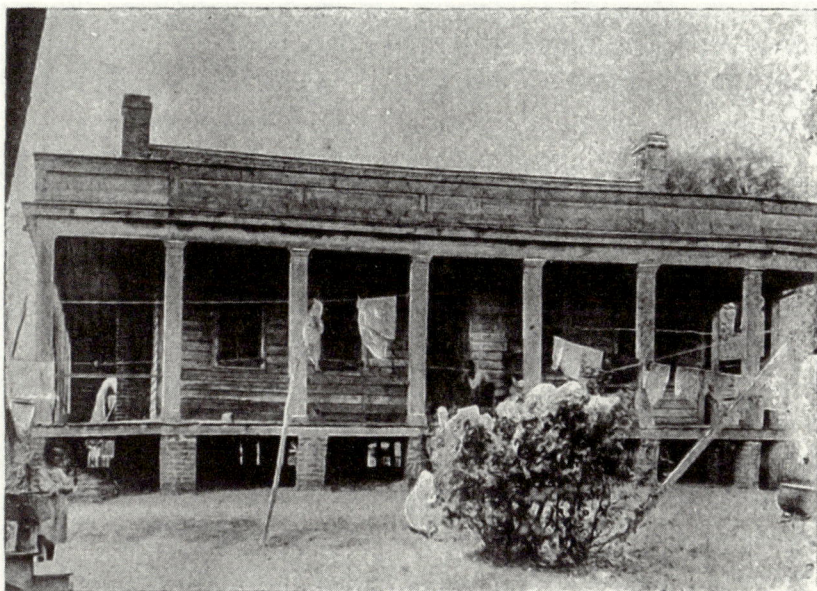

Dr. James Marion Sims's first women's hospital, Montgomery, Alabama (1895). Courtesy of Reynolds Historical Library, University of Alabama at Birmingham.

Georgia, plantation of Thomas Hamilton, a physician and trustee of the Medical Academy of Georgia. Brown eventually made his way to England, where in 1855, he told his story to the secretary of the British and Foreign Slavery Society. In minute detail, Brown recalled how Dr. Hamilton built a fire in a deep ditch and forced him to sit naked on a stool in the pit. Hamilton used a thermometer to judge Brown's endurance at different levels of heat. "Though I tried hard to keep up against its effects," Brown said, "in about half an hour I fainted. I was then lifted out and revived, the Doctor taking note of the degrees of heat when I left the pit." Following each day's work in the field, Brown repeated his ordeal with the heat in the open pit.[18]

Rising numbers of physicians advertised in newspapers in the South for the purchase of sick slaves for the purpose of experimenting with different surgical procedures. Thomas Hamilton, discussed above, may have purchased John Brown as a sick slave. Evidence suggests that he "cured Brown of a mysterious illness" but bought him to conduct "a great number of experiments" on his body designed to find a cure for "sunstroke." In May 1839, a Dr. King of New Orleans advertised in the city's *Picayune* for slaves with a list of specific ailments, especially "female diseases." In South Carolina, Dr. T. Sullivan "sought sick, disabled, diseased and nearly dead enslaved people" in an ad posted with the *Charleston Mercury*. "TO PLANTERS AND OTHERS," the ad stated. "Wanted *fifty negroes*. Any person having sick negroes, considered incurable by their respective physicians and wishing to dispose of them." The ad went on to specify that "Dr. S. will pay cash for negroes affected with scrofula or king's evil . . . diseases of the liver, kidneys, spleen, stomach and intestines, bladder and its appendages, diarrhea, [and] dysentery."[19]

Other physicians purchased sick slaves to cure and then place them back on the market at a higher price. With few exceptions, these were adult men and women. Slave traders, physicians, and owners routinely placed the health and well-being of infants and children at the bottom of their list of priorities in the buying and selling of humans. In the slaveholding pens prior to sale on the open market, children were most often "not treated at all and were quickly sold" once their parents were purchased, died, or removed from the pens.[20] For adults, however, the widespread search for "deceased" and nearly deceased people opened the door for the rise of a thriving trade in the cadavers of enslaved persons. The cadaver trade spread across the South and North during the early nineteenth century. In her influential book *The Price of Their Pound of Flesh*, historian Daina Ramey Berry documents the ways that deceased slaves acquired what she describes as "ghost value." Upon death, African American bodies were assigned a legal "price tag" as they "circulated through the domestic cadaver trade."[21]

Physicians, the medical profession, and medical schools represented the principal clients for dead bodies for experimentation to improve the health of white people. Anthropologists Robert L. Blakely and Judith M. Harrington succinctly captured this apparent paradox in racist medical science. "Although southern physicians of the nineteenth century held the same racist notions about the inferiority of blacks as the rest of southern society and went so far as to teach that blacks and whites differed anatomically, they nevertheless used black cadavers to teach medical students human anatomy and performed medical experiments on living black people to benefit mainly their white patients."[22] At a time when most states, North and South, prohibited the acquisition of dead bodies for medical experimentation, deceased African Americans became the principal suppliers of corpses (along with whites executed for capital offenses) for the nation's medical schools and physicians. Between the late eighteenth century and the mid-nineteenth century, students in US medical schools dissected over 4,000 bodies as part of their training to become recognized as professional physicians. Enslaved Blacks provided the vast majority of these cadavers—some acquired through the consent of slave owners and others secured through the underground economy of "grave-robbing" or "body-snatching." In one six-month period from September 1831 to February 1832, "grave-robbers" in Richmond, Virginia, "relieved" sixteen graves of their contents and delivered them to the University of Virginia Medical School in Charlottesville.[23] According to Berry, Southern cities like Richmond "harvested slave corpses" and prepared them for shipment replete with shipping rates as follows:

Adults—$12
14 years being considered adult age
Subjects from 4–10—$8
Mother and infant—$15
Infants from birth to 8 years—$4.[24]

There was a similar but smaller trade in enslaved and free Black residents of Northern cities. In New York City, both Columbia University and New York University secured bodies from the "Negroes Burying Ground." As early as 1788, African Americans petitioned the New York City Common Council to stop medical students from raiding the Black graveyard "under the cover of Night," mangling the flesh of the deceased, and leaving the bodies exposed "to the Beasts and Birds." One white newspaper justified the students' actions, arguing that "the only subjects procured for dissection are the productions of Africa . . . if these are the only subjects of dissection, surely no one can object."[25] Some of these Black bodies also found their way into cadaver commercial circuits that supplied medical schools in Southern cities. A New York provider of cadavers sold $100 worth of bodies to the Medical College of Georgia (Augusta) in 1839. Their shipment paralleled the transshipment of thousands of enslaved Blacks from the Upper South to the Deep South during the antebellum years. As Berry notes, the subjects were shipped "along the same routes as the shipments of living enslaved people."[26]

Claiming Expertise in the Treatment of Enslaved People:
Building a Plantation Clientele

At the same time that increasing numbers of physicians and medical schools sought Black bodies for their experiments and physician education programs, other aspiring doctors appealed to plantation owners' material investment in the creation and maintenance of an able-bodied Black enslaved labor force. They presented themselves as experts on the diagnosis and treatment of sick slaves and saw this service as a route to establish a viable livelihood for themselves and their families. These practitioners also embraced widespread notions about Black and white differences, presumably requiring alternative forms of specialized knowledge and treatment to effect successful cures. Rather than advertising to acquire sick bondmen and women for experimentation and education purposes, this set of physicians aimed to persuade planters to hire their services to help keep enslaved hands healthy and at work in the fields and households of their owners.

In her innovative study of health among the enslaved, medical historian Sharla M. Fett employed the term "soundness" to describe able-bodied labor, property, and profits at the center of slave owner interest in African American health and health care. The notion of "soundness" gained widespread articulation among the planters, physicians, and even African American commentators as the plantation economy expanded and consolidated around cotton production during the antebellum years.[27] In 1852, in the *Charleston Medical Journal*, the physician W. Fletcher Homes declared that the planter's "wealth consists chiefly in his negroes, and in proportion to their thrift and healthiness, just in such ratio does he prosper. The principal value of the negro with us is his increase, consequentially [slave health] addresses itself to the interest as well as the humanity of the slave-holder." Similarly, in 1849, the fugitive slave turned minister and abolitionist James W. C. Pennington described how the "being of slavery, its soul and body, lives and moves in the chattel principle." As such, Pennington expressed his strong conviction that the principle of "human property," "bill of sale," and the "soundness" idea governed the planter's interest in the slave's health and trumped all other considerations, human or material. According to Fett, the "intersection of medicine with the southern political economy produced a narrow definition of slave health permeated by concerns of slaveholder status and wealth" over the physical and mental well-being of the enslaved.[28]

South Carolina emerged as a major site of widespread advertisements geared toward selling medical services to urban and plantation slaveholders alike. James Clitherall, a low country physician loyal to the British Crown, returned to Charleston after departing the city in the wake of the American Revolution. He swiftly turned toward rebuilding his medical practice by advertising in the *South Carolina Gazette*, considered the city's first successful newspaper. His advertisements accented his capacity to meet the medical needs of enslaved workers, including dental care, midwifery, surgery, and even the provision of medicine for plantation residents and as well as ships plying the Atlantic and gulf ports.[29] Clitherall also announced his plans to build "a Hospital for the reception of Negroes, either in Clinical or Surgical Cases." In 1791, a Dr. Sheed advertised his plan to construct a "Hospital for the reception of sick negroes" in Charleston at 277 King Street between Tradd and Broad Street. A year later, another physician, listed only as Dr. Bartlett, advertised a hospital for "negroes laboring under diseases requiring medical or chirurgical assistance." Still another doctor, Haitian émigré L. Signeur, advertised in the *City Gazette and Daily Advertiser* that his "HOUSE OF HEALTH is now in the best order and ready to receive such SLAVES" that might "be entrusted" to his care.[30]

Motivated by a combination of self-interest for their own health and the health of their families, as well as a desire to protect their material investment in slave "property," some large well-endowed plantations and slaveholders slowly erected hospitals to serve the enslaved population before the beginning of the Civil War. These facilities were not only "separate from the main slave quarters," but they were also used to isolate slaves with "contagious diseases."

Planters were not moved to hire physicians entirely on their own volition. Beginning in the eighteenth century through the early nineteenth century, they became the target of vigorous advertising campaigns by newly trained physicians who sought to enter lucrative medical service agreements with plantation owners to serve the enslaved population. As historian Rana Hogarth notes, these physicians sought to carve out a living for themselves as health care professionals within the context of a society dominated by the highly profitable employment of enslaved African labor. In 1853, a Tennessee physician publicly argued, "Every plantation should be provided with a hospital. . . . There should always be two rooms, so that the sexes may be kept separate. . . . Single beds should be used, with good mattresses, and made comfortable as possible."[31]

Such rhetoric aimed to attract the attention of slave owners intent on preserving the health of their workforce. It did little to curtail the ways that racist medical science and physician practices undermined the health care of enslaved and free people of color across early America. The early medical profession expressed little to no interest in the emotional and spiritual well-being of African people. When it did, priority was given not to emotional recovery but to the restoration of the person's capacity to work. Rising numbers of medical professionals valued highly diseased or even deceased Black bodies over living ones for dissection and experimentation purposes. And what those laboratory parts revealed served the educational needs of the next generation of Euro-American medical practitioners. Such callous disregard for the health and well-being of enslaved people combined with the debilitating impact of staple crop labor and hazardous living conditions to imperil the health and well-being of Black people from the beginning of European settlement of North America through the onset of the Civil War.

The Health Consequences of Tobacco, Rice, and Sugar Production

Enslaved people cultivated an expanding range of lucrative but health-threatening staple crops against the backdrop of white supremacist ideas and practices in early American medicine, health care, politics, and society. Tobacco, rice, and sugar cultivation emerged at the center of the colonial economy, followed by the rise the "cotton kingdom" in the wake of the American Revolution and the rise of the new republic. In different ways, each of the staples resulted in damage to the health and well-being of enslaved African people. Tobacco agriculture, which was the primary staple for early Virginia and Maryland, required both strenuous labor and meticulous care. The planter John Carter described tobacco as "a very tender plant" that acquired a much deserved reputation as "a plant of perpetual trouble and difficulty."[32] As staple crop historians note, tobacco cultivation often strained "every nerve" of an enslaved worker's body. Cultivating tobacco not only severely strained the bodies of bondmen and women but also exposed them to specific occupational diseases. These were most pronounced in the preparation of the crop for market and in the tobacco factories that sprang up in proximity to the tobacco fields.[33]

The greatest health hazard of tobacco production involved lung disease caused by the constant inhalation of tobacco fumes. Tobacco bale "unloaders" and "unpackers" bore the brunt of dust inhalation. The dust also irritated the eyes, causing excessive tearing and damage to the sight of tobacco workers. Moreover, when the dust fumes mixed with juice from the tobacco leaves, it "caused rashes on the face and backs of hands." But all tobacco workers suffered from the constant inhalation of nicotine, including acute poisoning for some workers that resulted in insomnia, nausea, and vomiting. Furthermore, during the drying and stemming of tobacco for market "respirable-sized silica particles" caused "tobacosis," a lung disease similar to black lung among coal miners.[34]

Life, labor, and health challenges were even greater in the Lower South, where rice production predominated. During the early to mid-eighteenth century, South Carolina moved from a mixed economy of small farming and cattle-raising for the West Indian market to an increasing dependence on enslaved Africans who produced rice, which became integral to the economy of the South Carolina low country economy. One late 18th century observer, James Glen, remarked that, "The only Commodity of Consequence produced in *South Carolina is Rice* . . . and they reckon it as much their staple Commodity, as *sugar* is to *Barbados* and *Jamaica,* or Tobacco to *Virginia* and *Maryland."* Rice production accounted for 50 to nearly 70 percent of South Carolina's total value of exports during most of the colonial era. According to another eighteenth-century observer, "Rice is raised as to buy more negroes, and negroes are bought as to get more rice."[35]

A long and laborious process, rice cultivation took from twelve to fourteen months to complete from initial preparations to shipment to consumers in international trade networks. French historian Fernand Braudel compared the labor requirements of rice production with a variety of other crops and concluded that "rice holds the record for the man handling it requires."[36] According to historian Philip D. Morgan, "The rice cycle was the most arduous, the most unhealthy, and the most prolonged of all mainland staples."[37] In his popular poem *Carolina or, The Planter,* George Ogilvie likened the establishment and cultivation of rice plantations to the "rechanneling of the Euphrates and the building of the pyramids."[38] In order to construct an extensive network of "banks, canals, ditches, and drains," enslaved people regularly removed some 500 cubic yards of river swamp for each acre of rice under cultivation.

In their advertisements for enslaved workers, South Carolina planters sought labor for the special conditions of rice cultivation. The planter Pierce Butler advertised for "a gang of Negroes accustomed to Cultivate Rice." He made it clear that he wanted "no cotton negroes." He wanted only "people that can go in the Ditch."[39] Work in the ditch exposed Black people to a variety of "pleurises and lung diseases," including influenza, pneumonia, and tuberculosis. In the 1720s and again during the 1740s, South Carolina Governor James Glen reported that planters who invested in African labor might see their workforce "swept off" by lung disease "if not by smallpox."[40] Rice planters imported 15,000 new Africans between 1734 and 1740, but the Black population rose from about 26,000 to only 40,000 during the same period. This pattern resembled the Caribbean, where planters often "worked slaves to death" because they could rely on cheap sources of new workers from the transatlantic slave trade. Only slowly would new births exceed death rates for South Carolinians of African descent.[41]

A similarly harsh work environment greeted enslaved African people in the sugar producing low country of Louisiana. Nearly two decades after proprietors established South Carolina under the British Crown, the French claimed possession of the Louisiana Territory. During the 1720s, France initiated an aggressive drive to transform Louisiana into a colony growing tobacco, indigo, and finally sugar, with New Orleans as its center and using enslaved African labor.[42] The Haitian Revolution against French rule opened the door for other areas, including Louisiana, to compete for the lucrative sugar trade. When the United States acquired the Louisiana Territory in 1803, the colony produced over 4.5 million pounds of sugar valued at nearly a million dollars. By 1860, the fourteen largest sugar parishes reported 116,000 enslaved people who produced some "87,000 metric tons of sugar, along with cotton and corn." Sugar, as many commentators declared, "became king in lower Louisiana."[43]

From the outset of Louisiana's labor history, enslavement took a huge toll on the lives of African people. Early Africans built the levees and drainage ditches along the Mississippi River; they cleared forest land and cut and hauled timber for the construction of plantation houses and other buildings and ultimately constructed and toiled on large sugar plantations that produced increasing volumes of sugar that greatly enriched slaveholding elites. Much like the South Carolina rice region, sugar mortality rates were exceedingly high. Because of Louisiana's location well within the North American frost zone, sugar production was an extraordinarily precarious and intricate process that reinforced the imposition of an excessively harsh work regimen on the enslaved people. Compared to the Caribbean, Louisiana sugar growers had to harvest the crop some nine to ten months following the annual planting season whereas the crop actually required fourteen to eighteen months to mature. In a push to harvest ahead of the first frost, planters intensified pressure on enslaved men, women, and children.[44]

During the harvest season, enslaved workers toiled "sixteen or more hours a day, seven days a week." In 1833, during his visit to Louisiana, Thomas Hamilton, a British military officer, reported on the work regimen in the sugar region, observing that "the crop in Louisiana is never considered safe till it is in the mill, and the consequence is that when cutting once begins, the slaves are taxed beyond their strength, and are goaded to labour until nature absolutely sinks under the effort." In short, Hamilton emphatically concluded that sugar cultivation was carried out "at an enormous expense of human life." "Planters must buy," he said, "to keep up their stock, and this supply principally comes from Maryland, Virginia, and North Carolina."[45] In addition to carrying out all phases of field and maintenance work on the plantation, enslaved sugar workers performed "all the labor involved in processing the crop from feeding and stoking the mill to loading hogsheads of sugar and barrels of molasses onto the river steamers at the plantation wharf."[46]

The suffering of overworked, ill, and tortured sugar workers sometimes reached the colony's Superior Council. In 1727, one slave owner petitioned the council against his overseer "for ruining one of his most valuable slaves" as punishment for the offense of running away. The overseer had tightly bound the runaway's hands and given him "600 rawhide lashes." In the process of administering this extreme punishment, the enslaved man "lost two fingers from his right hand and two fingertips from his left hand." The Superior Council also heard the case of another "brutish overseer" who had regularly raped and tortured slave women "in the open field," withheld essential food provisions, and caused "frequent abortion among the slave women" by severe corporal punishment during pregnancy.[47] An estimated 7,000 Africans arrived in Louisiana between 1718 and 1735, but the resident African population stood at only 3,400 at the end of this period.[48] Into the early nineteenth century, the impact of sugar production on the health of the enslaved population continued to punctuate the day-to-day operations of the plantation economy. In August 1807, the slave owner Henry Brown reported that fifteen enslaved workers were sick "with a respiratory ailment and one woman had died." Yet Brown said, "I grow fat in spite of heat and fatigue . . . we (I mean my own family & self) continue thank God to enjoy fine health."[49]

In rice, sugar, and tobacco cultivation, the employment of enslaved African workers varied tremendously over time. But the system of human bondage culminated with the rapid spread of cotton production into the Deep South states during the early nineteenth century. The massive transport of some 1.5 million enslaved people from the Upper to Lower South also took a huge toll on the health of Black people. Planters who relocated to the Deep South regularly wrote back home about the sickness and death among the new African American arrivals to the cotton region.

Emergence of the Deep South Cotton Economy

Shortly after migrating to the Alabama Territory, the planter Israel Pickens reported the death of "a Negro girl Chainy a daughter of old Esther. . . . Her complaint was consumption [or tuberculosis]." Another planter John Minor wrote to his sister that "Illness had struck the place." Some twenty hands "were down," two had died, and "old Roy, a skilled artisan, had contracted a hip ailment that threatened to prevent him from ever working again."[50]

Because of the forced migration and the rise of the "cotton kingdom," planters regularly lamented the lost days of labor occasioned by sickness among the enslaved workforce. On the Hermitage Plantation near Savannah, the manager K. Washington Skinner informed owner Charles Manigault that sickness among the "negroes retards the progress of the work very much. Jimmy, Ben, William, Lilly & Phillis are the sick today, and some of them have been for several days." Similarly, in a letter to his daughter, the slave owner William Cain of North Carolina reported on one slave woman: "poor Jinny Kirkland is grunting [complaining] and will be of no possible use for months but to consume good." Poor slave health also engaged the attention of South Carolina planter Thomas Chaplin, who regularly wrote in his journal on the status of slave health on his place. At one point, in January 1849, he wrote, "Moll taken to her bed with fever. This sickness is bad for me in getting out my crop." On another occasion, he wrote, "Isaac & Moll still sick. God knows when I will get all of my small force at work." At another moment, in January 1856, he reported, "Sancho sick, therefore one gin stopped."[51]

Although sugar, rice, and tobacco claimed the bulk of enslaved African labor before the onset of the American Revolution, cotton dominated African American life and labor during the early nineteenth century. Black people not only endured the painful forced migration from the Upper to the Lower South. They were also put to work building the cotton plantations before they could plant the first seeds, cultivate, and harvest the cotton crop. Enslaved workers carved out the cotton plantation from the earth and wilderness with backbreaking labor, "cutting trees, grubbing out and burning underbrush, constructing cabins, outbuildings, and fences," among a variety of other tasks ahead of cotton production.[52]

Cotton required extensive plowing, hoeing, and picking, and like the other staples grown across the region, the strict supervision of overseers armed with the power of the lash or whip.[53] Most overseers and drivers used a narrow strip of tough cowhide, whipcord, or cat-o'-nine-tails, which left deep gashes in the skin. In his pioneering study *Medicine and Slavery*, historian Todd L. Savitt declared, "From a medical point of view, whipping inflicted cruel and often permanent injuries upon its victims. Laying stripes across the bare back or buttocks caused indescribable pain, especially when each stroke dug deeper into previously opened wounds."[54] More recently, Edward Baptist describes how severe floggings undermined the capacity of people to "speak in sentences or think coherently. They 'danced,' trembled, babbled, [and] lost control of their bodies." Nonetheless, driven by an unquenchable thirst for profits, slave owners consistently disputed the damage inflicted by the overseer's whip. "Sure, it might etch deep gashes in the skin of its victim, make them 'tremble' or 'dance' . . . but it did not disable them, enslavers reasoned." But the larger meaning of profits and the lash were not lost on African Americans. Henry Bibb, an ex-slave on a plantation along the Red River, later recalled how cotton planters produced large "quantities of cotton" and "extorted" their wealth "by the lash."[55]

Violence and coerced labor through regular use of the whip virtually erased differences in health and well-being from crop to crop. Nor were whippings restricted by gender and type of work. Although male field hands endured the most brutal torture through whippings, women and household workers were not immune. The whipping of slave women, as historian Deborah Gray White notes, carried sharp "sexual overtones." An escaped slave living in Canada, Christopher Nichols, "remembered how his master laid a woman on a bench, threw her clothes over her head, and whipped her." Another ex-slave described a whipping where the woman's naked "quivering" body was "tied up" and put on display for "the public gaze of all."[56]

Poor housing, improper clothing, inadequate diets, and unsanitary living conditions reinforced the health hazards of work environments. Pork was considered "King of the Table" among food provided for the enslaved population. The standard fare included a half pound of pork and one and a half pounds of corn or cornmeal. Most antebellum authorities believed that this diet provided some 4,000 to 6,000 calories per day, sufficient for long and hard hours of physical field labor. Recent scholarship on the subject suggests that even when supplemented somewhat by molasses, sweet potatoes, and diverse vegetable crops, most slave diets were insufficient to provide "resistance to most major diseases."[57]

The spread of deadly diseases intensified during the winter months when Blacks inhabited poorly ventilated and unhealthy quarters.[58] Whereas planters, small farmers, and poor whites lived in widely scattered rural households, Blacks often occupied dense three-, ten-, or thirty-family communities. Although planters clothed their personal servants and household workers in the best garments, they usually cut costs in dressing the field hands. Some scholars suggest that enslaved people were more prone to thermal injuries in cold rather than hot weather. During the winter, planters frequently complained that "Myself & several of the colored people have bad colds," or "Hands & children have suffered very much from colds-in fact cold has been quite an epidemic." But enslaved people worked indoors and outdoors year-round in all kinds of weather. Heat injuries were also substantial. In 1825, the owner of one Virginia plantation reported the "hottest day ever felt — men gave out some fainted." Intestinal diseases increased during the summer months, when people spent more time outdoors in direct contact with the earth.

Improper management of human waste and contaminated water also led to epidemics of cholera, dysentery, diarrhea, typhoid, and hepatitis, as well as influenza, pneumonia, tuberculosis, and diphtheria. A Richmond physician later recalled how the accumulated piles of human waste were "regularly [but not often enough] scraped up, and hauled off to enrich the land" as "night soil."[59] Enslaved people usually entered "the open air for the calls of nature, in all kinds of weather." Whether during the winter or summer, enslaved people faced the ravages of intestinal parasites that affected lungs, liver, blood vessels, gall bladder, vagina, anus, and skin. Worm infections included "tapeworms," associated with eating poorly cooked meat; "roundworms," associated with poor sanitation; and "hookworms," which entered the body through contact with the ground. Barefoot, field workers and ditch diggers were especially vulnerable to the hookworm. Enslaved plantation bound workers and their families also suffered from sexually transmitted diseases, mainly syphilis and gonorrhea; various types of tumors, especially those afflicting the skin and bones; and mental illness, described as "fits of insanity," "deranged," and "lunatic" slaves.[60]

Urban Industrial Context

The medical challenges of enslaved people were by no means limited to the plantation and farms of the agricultural South. Supplemented by a gradually expanding population of free people of color, African people also faced enslavement in colonial and early American cities of the North and South. Slave labor fueled the rise of Southern lumber, naval stores, coal, railroad, textile, tobacco, and iron companies. By 1860, hundreds of enslaved Blacks cut, loaded, and transported hardwood, cypress, oak, and pine to sawmills, where they not only hauled, stacked, and loaded finished slabs for transport to market but fired and operated the steam engines. Specific occupational hazards compounded the medical difficulties of industrial bondmen: lung disease afflicted tobacco workers; rock falls, deadly gases, and explosions injured and killed miners; and hot molten metal burned and damaged the skin and eyes of ironworkers.[61]

Enslaved and free Black women shouldered the twin burdens of reproductive and productive labor. The vast majority of mistresses used enslaved women "not as their personal attendant" but rather as heavy-laden domestic laborers—Black women were "put to work sweeping, emptying chamber pots, carrying water, washing the dishes, brewing, looking after children, cooking and baking, spinning, knitting, carding, and sewing."[62] Household labor not only entailed long hours and this tedious work—or whatever employers demanded—it also made Black women vulnerable to widespread physical and sexual abuse. In Charleston, some slave owners realized a "superordinate level of accumulation" by forcing enslaved women household workers to perform "sexual acts for money" in addition to their washing, cleaning, and other domestic tasks.[63]

Black urbanites, enslaved and free, lived and labored under even more congested and unsanitary conditions than their rural brothers and sisters. When one Virginia slave owner moved his family and enslaved Blacks from the farm to a house in town, over twenty Blacks died, as well as a few of his own family members. According to a report of the man's friend, crowded and unsanitary conditions precipitated the epidemic: "The lot was small, and back yard so much crowded with out houses, and trees, as to exclude the sun almost entirely. The cellars of course must have been exceedingly damp, and in them the Negroes lodged."[64]

Yellow fever, malaria, and cholera epidemics also took their toll on the lives of enslaved, free Blacks, and whites. Cholera resulted from humans drinking water contaminated from inadequate disposal of human waste. Hence, a virus led to infection. However, yellow fever and malaria were transmitted by mosquitoes; a parasite was transferred from the insect to the human, causing illness. Yellow fever epidemics broke out in Philadelphia in 1699, 1747, 1762, 1793, 1794, and 1798; in New York, Baltimore, Boston, New Haven, and New Orleans between 1793 and 1806; and in New Orleans in 1796. In their two-volume study of Black health care, W. Michael Byrd and Linda Clayton summarized the impact of yellow fever on victims bluntly but succinctly: "Half the susceptible victims vomit themselves to death over several days. Survivors are immune for life."[65] Environmental sociologist Dorceta E. Taylor offers a more elaborate account of the trajectory of the disease:

The more severe form of the disease characterized by the abrupt onset of shaking chills, fever, muscle aches, chilly fits, quick tense pulse, hot skin, headache, inflamed eyes, moist tongue, sore stomach, especially with applied pressure, and dark stool. This is followed by jaundice, creating a yellowish-purple tinge to the body, as the virus invades the liver, liver failure, and delirium . . . failure of the blood to clot results in hemorrhaging from the gums, nose, and stomach lining. This causes victims to vomit black blood. . . . Victims stop defecating and urinating and the kidneys fail. Death ensues about a day or two after renal failure, within a week of the onset of symptoms.[66]

We know much more about the Philadelphia yellow fever epidemic of 1793 than we know about the outbreak of the disease elsewhere. Although the Philadelphia epidemic took the lives of an estimated 4,000 whites and 250 Blacks, initially white residents insisted that the disease did affect people of African descent. The disease first broke out in New York City in 1703 and continued to recur through the early nineteenth century. When the fever hit New York City in 1801, 1803, and 1807, as historian Dorceta Taylor notes, "the myth persisted that blacks were immune to the disease." Similar to Philadelphia, elite whites, merchants, and others fled the city for the countryside, leaving behind "the poor classes and the negroes," whom they claimed were not "affected by the fever."

Such scenes played out in other cities as yellow fever broke out across the nation. Between 1832 and 1858, cholera broke out in New York City, Chicago, Cincinnati, and New Orleans. Among the major US cities, only Boston and Charleston escaped the ravages of cholera epidemics during the period. Cholera was a swift killer of its victims: "The onset of cholera is marked by diarrhea, vomiting, convulsions, and cramps. This causes dehydration, cyanosis, and cold and darkened extremities. As much as 35 percent of the body's fluids and up to 30 percent of body weight may be lost in a matter of hours. The symptoms appear without warning, and victims die within hours of the appearance of the first symptoms." In 1832, cholera took the lives of over 3,500 people, including Blacks and whites, in New York City.

Although the sickle cell trait provided immunity to malaria infection for large numbers of African people, malaria epidemics presented a recurring health challenge for enslaved and free people of color. A parasitic disease caused by the invasion of the red blood cells by a "one-celled animal" called "plasmodium," malaria infected large numbers of enslaved people in the plantation South. The initial onset of malaria is characterized by a spell of excessive chills. The chills cannot be abated "even by large numbers of blankets." Malaria was also, as historian Todd Savitt makes clear, "endemic throughout most of the slave South" rather than an episodic disease; "it posed a constant threat to health year in and year out, weakening the stricken so that other diseases often killed them." As Dr. Daniel Drake, a Southern physician and medical professor put it, the fevers "return every year in the latter part of summer and in autumn, and one attack is no security against another. When they do not prove fatal, they [nonetheless] leave behind them diseases of the spleen, and dropsy. In the following winter those [who] were down in the autumn, are tender, and often die of inflammation of the lungs." Following the chills are "extremely high fever, frequent nausea, vomiting, and severe headache."[67]

The repeated outbreaks of deadly epidemics compelled municipal authorities to gradually embrace reforms designed to "safeguard public health" across class and racial lines. Following the lead of Boston after its bout with the yellow fever epidemic in 1799, increasing numbers of cities established boards of health to help clean up the physical environment and safeguard the health of urban residents. While public health reforms helped to ease the plight of some urbanites suffering from a variety of diseases, they also more often reinforced class and racial inequalities in the health care system. Urban reforms and reformers heightened class discrimination against the white poor and reinforced the impact of racial inequality for Blacks.

Powerful elites advanced the notion that catastrophic diseases that took the lives of large numbers of urban residents were products of the immorality of the poor, Blacks as well as whites. In their view, the "immoral" life styles of the poor "weakened their constitution" and made them susceptible to deadly diseases. While these views led elite reformers to focus attention on cleaning up the city and creating more healthy physical environments for all residents, the moral component of their beliefs led them to embrace austere social welfare policies for the poor. As they moralized about the causes of disease, charities and relief committees severely curtailed aid to the poor and avoided making cash payment to people in need. They also intensified their oversight of the behavior of the poor before and after they dispensed aid.[68]

As class-biased social policies reinforced barriers to adequate health care for poor and working-class people across the color divide, the intensification of demeaning racial stereotypes against Blacks across class lines heightened indifference and neglect of African American health needs. Such neglect, however, was by no means entirely uniform over time or from place to place.

At the same time, across the antebellum South, small groups of physicians developed a tier of small private hospitals to serve the medical needs of enslaved and free people of color on a "for fee" basis. These facilities promised to provide board and lodging as well as medical care. Founded in 1832 in Savannah, the Georgia Infirmary promised "relief and protection of aged and afflicted Africans." It was considered the first private hospital created by whites to care for Blacks. The facility had "an endowment" to provide medical care for indigent free Blacks, but plantation owners had to pay for the treatment of their slaves. During the 1850s, also in Savannah, three white doctors opened another infirmary to treat "negroes requiring medical and surgical" services. The facility also offered patients maternity care, but it barred patients with "contagious diseases." This infirmary also advertised itself as a "well-appointed establishment" with "competent nurses, comfortable beds, well-ventilated wards, extensive pleasure grounds, and good food." Another antebellum medical institution, the Mississippi State Hospital, served slaves only and "charged their owners a dollar a day" for its work. In 1851, in Norfolk, Virginia, a group of physicians advertised the opening of an "Infirmary for Slaves" in a house "near Calvert's Lane," noting that "the location is private and central, and the house airy, well arranged and sufficiently commodious."[69]

Although hospitals and infirmaries serving the Black population were highly touted by planters, proslavery activists, and physicians as evidence of benign interest in the health and welfare of the enslaved and, to some extent, free people of color, such institutions proved woefully inadequate to address the suffering of the vast majority of enslaved workers, free people of color, and their families. Most medical institutions excluded African Americans in the North as well as the South. Northern Blacks were either denied treatment or served almost exclusively in "segregated wards," most often in "unheated attics or damp basements." In Philadelphia, at the Pennsylvania Hospital, physicians openly resisted serving wards with Black patients, especially those suffering from contagious disease. At about the same time, a foreign visitor reported his observation of the Louisville, Kentucky, City Hospital. He observed "roomy and well aired apartments for the white patients, and in the basement, those for the Negroes and colored persons."[70]

Postbellum activist newspaper editor Ida B. Wells captured the narrow self-interested and economic approach to antebellum Black health and health care. She described enslavement of Black people as a system that aimed "to dwarf the soul" but preserve the body of Black people to labor on behalf of their owners.[71] Moreover, even as rising numbers of slave owners hired resident physicians, many remained highly skeptical of the value of hiring their own doctors to attend to the enslaved workforce. In 1836, in Huntsville, Alabama, one owner of some 300 enslaved African Americans apparently fired his slave physician, arguing that "it was cheaper to lose a few negroes every year than pay a physician."[72] Hence, as most slave owners paid scant attention to the medical needs of Black people, African Americans organized their own health services. Their health activism resulted in the rise of dynamic plantation and, to some extent, urban-based Black systems of health care by the late antebellum years. These efforts were nonetheless closely in-tertwined with the spread of plantation owner- and white physician-led medical care among enslaved people.

Building Their Own Health Care System

Across eighteenth- and early nineteenth-century America, enslaved African people "took medical matters into their own hands." They were determined to establish their own health care system and break dependence on planta-tion medicine. Their strategies for improving their own health and the health of their families and communities included the fight for their own land to produce subsistence crops and supplement their diets; insistence on better treatment at work; and the gradual creation of formal social welfare, health, and mutual benefit organizations. Most important, however, enslaved people built on their African medical heritage. They challenged the market values of racial capitalism and advanced their own communal conceptualization of disease, health, and healing. As early as 1731 to 1812, African American heal-ers and medical practitioners had emerged across late colonial and early America, especially in the South. Their numbers included a broad range of "self-trained or informally trained" midwives, root doctors, and skilled herb-alists whose botanical knowledge was highly valued among slaveholders.[73] As such, enslaved rural African Americans not only influenced their own health but also shaped the larger system of plantation healing among white Southerners.[74]

Forging an African American Medical Practice

Building upon their West African medical heritage, beliefs, and practices, enslaved healers claimed the ability to both "harm and heal." According to historian and specialist on African American religious practices, Albert Rabo-teau, African people refused to "dichotomize power into good and evil." To paraphrase one Georgia woman, the conjurers and healer could both "cure and kill you." During the mid-1840s, on one Virginia plantation, an ill slave woman Patience rejected the white physician's diagnosis of her illness as "rheumatism." According to a letter to the woman's owner, written presum-ably by the overseer in charge of day-to-day work, "She thinks that she is tricked [or conjured] and desire a negro Doctor" to find a cure. The overseer rejected the woman's plea for alternative treatment and diagnosis, pre-scribing instead a bareback whipping as a cure. White physicians worked mightily to discredit the medical knowledge and practices of enslaved people. Mildred Graves, one plantation midwife later recalled how she was summoned to the bedside of a white woman to assist with a complicated birth. When she arrived, she found two white doctors already at the woman's side. When she told the physicians that she understood the woman's problem, they laughed and told her in no uncertain terms to stand back, "we mean business an' don' won't any witch doctors or hoo doo stuff." But the laboring woman soon "sent the white doctors away and retained Graves, who successfully delivered the baby."[75]

In some cases, European physicians took instructions from enslaved people to help remedy certain ailments. In colonial Louisiana, an African doctor taught one French physician (referred to as Le Page) his "secret cure for yaws and scurvy." Le Page later credited the Black doctor with imparting this knowledge: "The negro who taught me those remedies, observing the great care I took of both the negro men and negro women, taught me likewise the cure of all distempers to which the women are subject; for the negro women are as liable to disease as the white women." Similarly, in 1729, Lieutenant Governor William Gooch of Virginia liberated an enslaved man for "revealing his secret cure for venereal disease and yaws." Furthermore, Gooch said, "For the sake of his freedom, he has revealed the medicine, a concoction of roots and bark . . . it is well worth the price £60 of the negro's freedom, since it is now known how to cure slaves without mercury."[76]

Perhaps the earliest Black healer to gain widespread public notice was the fugitive slave Simon. In 1740, the *Pennsylvania Gazette* reported on Simon's escape from human bondage. The fugitive claimed to be "a great doctor among his people" with skills "to bleed and draw teeth." By 1748, the number of Blacks identifying themselves as doctors by occupation had proliferated, all claiming knowledge "to procure and prepare poisons" to both heal the sick and punish "their masters or enemies, both black and white." As the numbers of such doctors multiplied, Virginia legislators enacted a statute to "prohibit all slaves, on pain of death, from administering medicines without the consent of the owners of both the 'doctor' and the prospective black patient." In 1792, however, no doubt reflecting ongoing Black resistance to the law, the legislature amended the measure to permit the acquittal of enslaved Blacks who "administered medicines with good intentions, provided the drugs had caused patients no harm."

Some planters recognized that enslaved doctors provided better and more effective treatment for certain illnesses than the white plantation doctor. The enslaved people themselves also pushed planters to bring in their fellow slave doctors. Robert Carter, a Virginia planter, reported sending one of his slaves, named Guy, to the plantation of William Berry of King George County to receive treatment from Berry's slave named David. Guy had been languishing for some eighteen months without much improvement when Carter decided to send him to David. But it was Guy who pushed his owner to make that decision. In his correspondence, Carter noted how Guy was "very desirous of becoming a Patient of Negroe David." Carter then revealed how he consented to Guy "going up to yr house to be under the care & direction of David." The planter expected to leave the sick man in charge of David for several days in order for David to "observe the operation of the first [dose of] medicine" and prescribe the "appropriate drugs" for his recovery. Carter had also owned another enslaved man, Tom, a coachman, who gained a substantial reputation as a healer, treating enslaved people "throughout the neighborhood" in the 1770s. According to one contemporary white observer, "the Black people at this place [Taurus farm] hath more faith in him [Tom] as a Doctor than any white Doctr."[77]

During the nineteenth century, evidence of the workings of the internal slave medical system is even more abundant than for earlier times. As the American-born Black population increased, rising numbers of enslaved healers interacted with, influenced, and learned from Euro-American physicians. As suggested previously, African and African American healers interacted with Euro-American and European doctors from the outset of the transatlantic slave trade. The earliest Black doctor to claim expertise in bleeding and drawing teeth emerged in the early eighteenth century, but Black "leechers and cuppers or tooth-pullers" apparently increased in the new republic. In 1844, the Richmond slave owner John Walker hinted at the expanding African American medical network in a letter to James Sims, a free Black cooper. Sims wanted to hire Walker's enslaved man Daniel to assist him in his work. Walker agreed but gave Sims strict instructions on the treatment of Daniel should he become ill, "In the case of sickness you must employ [the white] Docr. Robinson to attend Daniel as I am not disposed to employ a Colored Docr to attend him." This letter suggests that without such explicit instructions, Sims would have turned to the network of Black physicians should Daniel require medical care. In Richmond, one resident humorously described a father-son team who practiced both dentistry and surgery:

Now-a-days the profession of dentry gives lucrative employment in our city to a score of practitioners. In the days of my boyhood, only one

Tooth-drawer, who probably never hear the word dentist, did all the work and all the mischief in the dental line.

Peter Hawkins was tall, raw-boned, very black negro who rode a raw-boned, black horse, for his practice was too extensive to manged on foot, and he carried all his instruments, consisting of two or three pullikins, in his pocket. His dexterity was such that he has been known to be stopped in the street by one of his distressed brethren, (for he was of the church), and to relieve him of the offending tooth, gratuitously, without dismounting from his horse. His strength of wrist was such that he would almost infallibly extract, or break a tooth, whether the right or the wrong one. I speak from sad experience, for he extracted two for me, a sound and an aching one, with one wrench of his instrument.

On Sundays he mounted the pulpit instead of black barebones, and as a preacher he drew the fangs of Satan with his spiritual pullikins, almost as skillfully as he did the teeth of his brother sinners on week days, with his metallic ones.

Peter's surgical, but not his clerical mantle, fell on his son, who depletes the veins and pockets of his patients, and when he has exhausted the latter, the former are respited. The doctor dismisses himself, and as likely as not, carries the malady with him.[78]

Black Women Healers

Black health providers, especially Black women, sometimes served "all ranks of society from the richest whites to the poorest blacks." African American women became the principal givers of "prenatal and obstetrical care of whites and blacks." African American women, as nurses and midwives, constituted the critical backbone of both plantation medicine and the Black network of self-help medicine. Midwives helped to deliver most babies born across the rural antebellum South. These women existed on every plantation, and they practiced throughout the neighborhoods of their areas. During the 1930s, one ex-slave midwife recalled her wide-ranging services to Black and white women in Hanover County, Virginia. Like many skilled midwives, she was also hired out on a regular basis. As she recalled in her own words:

> You know in dem days dey didn't have so many doctors. So treatin' de sick was always my mob. Whenever any of de white folks's 'roun' Hanover was goin' to have babies dey always got word to Mr. Tinsley dat day want tohire me for dat time. Sho' he lef me go . . .'twas money

for him, you know. He would give me only a few cents, but dat was kinda good of him to do dat. Plenty n . . . . . s was hired out an' didn't get nothin'. Sometimes I had three an' four sick at de same time, Marser used to tell me I was valuable slave. Dey use to come for me both day an's night—you know it's a funny thing how babies has a way comin' heah when it's dark.[79]

During the 1820s, the enslaved woman Jennifer Snow became "a living legend" in Petersburg, Virginia, for her "nursing and curative skills." On January 15, 1825, Snow's owner Benjamin Harrison manumitted her for providing "several acts of extraordinary merit performed . . . during the last year, in nursing, & at the imminent risk of her own health & safety, exercising the most unexampled patience and attention in watching over the sick beds of several individuals of this town." Harrison further expressed his "belief and desire" that Snow "continue, whenever occasion shall require to perform similar acts equally meritorious & praiseworthy." After receiving her freedom, Snow established her own hospital and offered her services to the community over the next three decades. Thirty years later, a local newspaper reported on operations performed by physicians "at the hospital of the well known nurse, Jincey Snow."

Despite the horrors of violent experimentation on Black bodies, in rare cases the results seemed salutary for some bondmen and women. As early as 1809, for example, Ephraim McDowell, a physician in Danville, Kentucky, reported the successful removal of a fifty-pound ovarian tumor from a forty-five-year-old Black woman who then reportedly went on to live for another twenty-five years. On another occasion when Abraham, an enslaved Charleston man, suffered a hernia that resulted in "a grossly enlarged genital area," his owner sent for a skilled white surgeon to correct the problem. The physician "performed an amputation of the middle section of Abraham's penis and sewed the ends together." Following three months of recovery, the physician reported that Abraham had carried out successful sexual "communication with a woman." Some enslaved women acquired extraordinary medical knowledge as nurses for physicians performing such operations. While Harriet Washington emphasized the unethical and painful practice of employing female slaves for medical experimentation, historian Deirdre Cooper Owens accented the way enslaved women—Anarcha, Betsy, Lucy, and about nine other enslaved women and girls—"worked together in the slave hospital that Dr. James Marion Sims founded for his own training and for the surgical repair of his patients."[80]

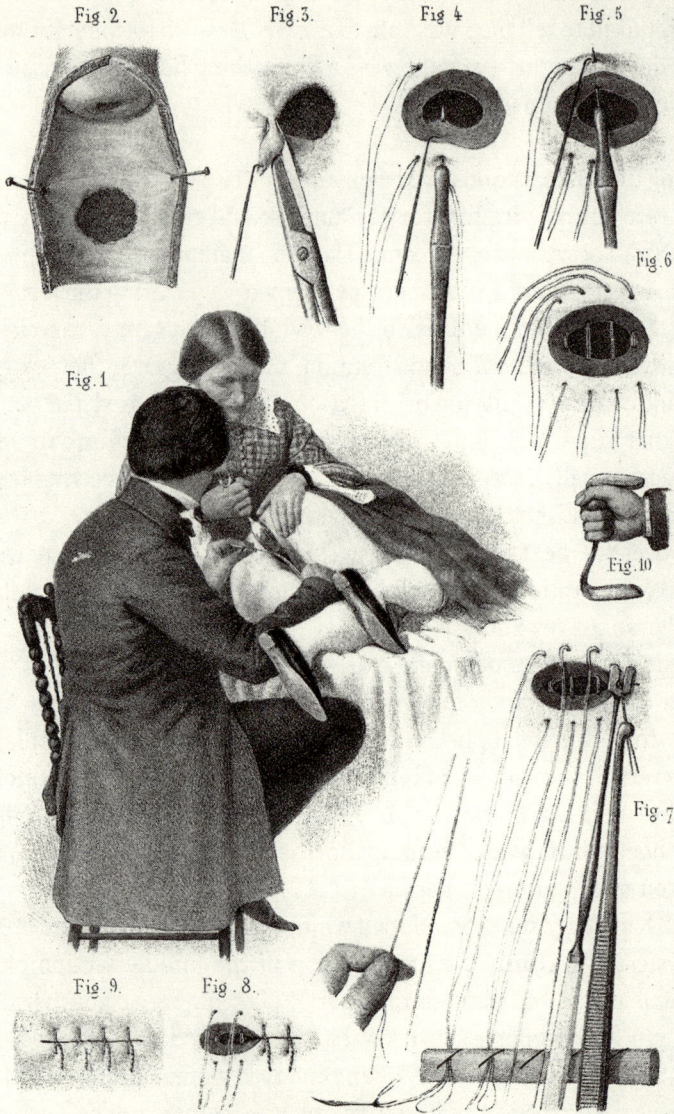

Surgical instruments and surgery performed by Dr. James Marion Sims and nurse. Reprinted from Henry Savage, *The Surgery, Surgical Pathology, and Surgical Anatomy of the Female Pelvic Organs* (London: John Churchill & Sons, 1862).

According to Cooper Owens, following recuperation from surgery, the women Sims operated on "continued to perform the duties slaves were expected to complete," including assisting Sims as "surgical nurses." In their capacity as "surgical nurses," Cooper Owens firmly argued that these women helped Sims "give birth" to the new medical field of gynecology. In her view, "enslaved women knew more about the repair of obstetrical fistulae than most American doctors during the mid-to late 1840s." In short, they helped to establish and run the "first women's hospital in the United States" between 1844 and 1849. Other widely known Black nurses during the antebellum years included abolitionists and antislavery activists Sojourner Truth (1797–1881) and Harriet Tubman (1820–1913). Both Truth and Tubman used their nursing skills to care for "wounded civilians and soldiers" during the Civil War.[81]

Gaining Access to Western Medical Training

In addition to a network of independent self-trained or informally trained medical doctors and nurses, an exceptional few African Americans received formal medical education at elite universities at home and abroad. As early as the 1660s, in New Netherlands, Lucas Santomee, a Dutch-trained Black physician, practiced medicine in the first two buildings constructed on Manhattan Island to serve "sick soldiers and Negroes." Santomee became "well-known in the colony as a physician." But no other university-trained Black physicians appeared during the colonial era or the United States until the early nineteenth century, when James McCune Smith (1813–65) received an MD degree from the University of Glasgow in Scotland in 1837.[82]

Between the 1830s and the onset of the Civil War, a significant but exceedingly small coterie of university-trained Black physicians emerged in the United States. In addition to James McCune Smith, this tiny cohort of early nineteenth-century Black doctors included most notably David John Peck, John Rock, and Martin Delany, among a few others. Born in New York City to an ex-slave father and free mother, Smith received his primary education at the New African Free School established by the New York Manumission Society. When he returned to New York after earning his MD degree, he set up a lucrative medical practice and "opened two highly regarded apothecary shops." Smith also established a model for providing both health services and civil rights advocacy for the African American community.

Subsequent Black physicians would seek to emulate the work of James MCune Smith. As one medical historian put it, Smith "set a pattern generally followed ever since: he became a leader of his people, and was an

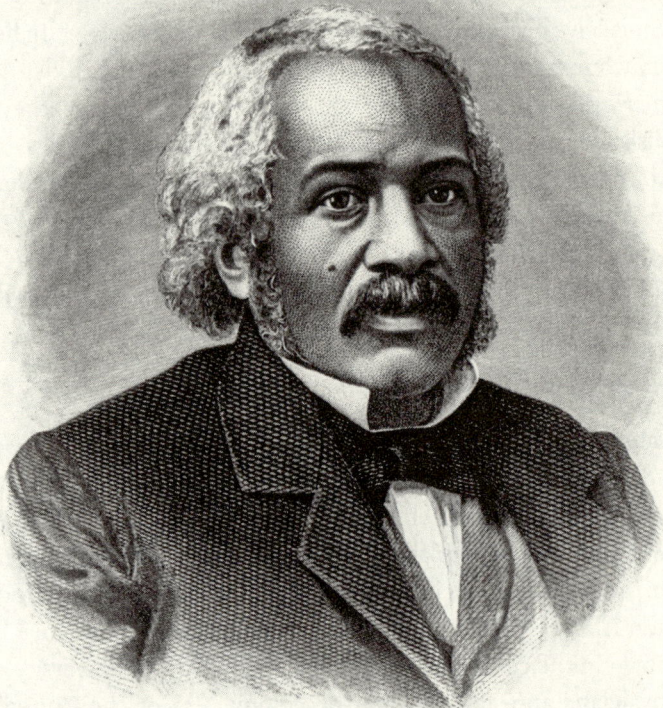

Engraved by Patrick H Reason

James McCune Smith

Engraving of Dr. James McCune Smith, MD (1811–65), health activist and first African American to earn a formal medical degree from the University of Glasgow, Scotland, in 1837. Reprinted from W. Michael Byrd and Linda Clayton, *An American Health Dilemma: A Medical History of African Americans and the Problem of Race, Beginnings to 1900* (New York: Routledge, 2000). Courtesy of the New York Historical Society.

ardent abolitionist." Smith not only diligently served the health needs of New York City's Black community, but he also waged an ongoing fight against racism in the medical profession. In 1844, in a "Memorial to the U.S. Senate," he refuted "the racist use of the fraudulent U.S. Census by the Secretary of State, John C. Calhoun." Supported by a sympathetic white ally, Dr. Edward Jarvis, as well as his own careful statistical review of the data, Smith was able to reveal how the census returned some towns and cities without any Black residents as having so many "insane negroes." As Jarvis put it, "So far from being an aid to medical science, it had thrown a stumbling block in its ways, which will require years to remove."[83]

In 1840, for the first time, the Sixth Census of the United States enumerated whites and free and enslaved Blacks. It also counted "insane and idiots" in the population. These were the terms regularly used during the period to identify the mentally ill and intellectually challenged. But the 1840 Census, published by the US Department of State, contained numerous errors based on deliberate and racially biased use of statistics and the tools of the emerging science of quantitative analysis. The report included mounds of tables replete with figures on the health status of Black people. On virtually every measure of well-being, including disease, infant mortality, death and birth rates, free people of color, particularly in the urban North, fared worse than the enslaved Black population in the South. The report gave defenders of slavery and slaveholding a major intellectual resource for resisting the abolitionist movement. Based on the 1840 Census, proslavery Southerners repeatedly argued that emancipation would result in the extinction of the Black race. On US letterhead, Calhoun had spread the proslavery message of the 1840 Census across America and overseas.[84]

David John Peck, another early nineteenth-century Black physician, was the first African American to receive an MD degree from a US medical school. Born in Pittsburgh, Peck was a friend of the physician, abolitionist, and Black nationalist Martin R. Delany (1812–1885). He enrolled in the Rush Medical College in Chicago, after facing numerous obstacles gaining admission to other medical schools. Peck faced equally daunting barriers to his effort to establish a viable medical practice after receiving his medical degree. He then joined one of Delany's emigration projects in Nicaragua in Central America. In Nicaragua, he was soon named Port physician and developed "a booming practice" and was appointed to a "high post in the government" of the country.

For his part, Martin Delany, described by Byrd and Clayton as "Black Medicine's Spartacus," was born in Charles Town, West Virginia, and moved with his family to Pittsburgh by the 1820s. He received apprentice training in medicine from some of the city's leading white physicians, including the abolitionist F. Julius Le Moyne. Delany also took courses at a variety of medical schools, including Harvard. Whether he graduated from any of these institutions, however, is still a subject of debate. In any case, his interest in the medical profession increasingly gave way to his growing involvement in the global struggle to liberate African people within and beyond the shores of North America. He became one of the foremost emigrationists among early nineteenth-century African Americans, but he also consistently challenged racism in the medical profession. He left an indelible mark on the African American struggle to demolish the racial underpinnings of modern medical science. According to Byrd and Clayton, Delany "openly debated white politicians and scientists and debunked the myth of Black biological and racial inferiority." During the Civil War, Delany would distinguish himself as "an officer and surgeon" in the Union Army.

A Delaney contemporary and a polymath, John Sweat Rock gained prominence for his legal work on behalf of the African American community. In December 1865, he became the first African American to gain certification to practice law at the US Supreme Court, but his medical career preceded that achievement. Rock earned his MD degree from the Medical College of Philadelphia. Before that, he had apprenticed and gained formal training in dentistry as well as medicine. Ultimately, he decided to set up a dental rather than medical practice among African Americans in Philadelphia. As a result of declining health brought on by tuberculosis, however, he abandoned his dental practice and entered the field of law. After being named the first African American to practice law before the nation's highest court, he died of tuberculosis just over a year later. Despite his short sojourn in the medical field, Rock's life illuminated the substantial role that a tiny group of formally trained Black physicians played in the health care and medical history of the African American community. It comprised an integral part of the emerging antebellum Black health care system.[85]

Land, Institutions, and the Fight for Better Health

The struggle against medical apartheid was not limited to the development of a subsystem of Black health care providers. It also included the quest for land not only as a route to independence, freedom, and empowerment but also for the production of foodstuffs to offset the imbalanced slave diet, improve their health, and expand their life expectancy. Some scholars suggest that the African American lifespan gradually increased over the long eighteenth century but came to an end during the second decade of the nineteenth century, before gradually rising again thereafter. But the gap between Black and white longevity persisted through the Civil War and emancipation era. By the late nineteenth century, Black men lived on average about thirty to thirty-two years, while Black women lived slightly longer about thirty-four years. But their white counterparts lived fifty years or more. Considered the "gold standard" of health status and outcomes, available life expectancy data show that African Americans registered considerably below their white brothers and sisters before and after slavery.

From the outset of their sojourn in North America, bondmen and women developed a keen sense of property ownership and insisted on access to their own plots of land not only to serve their health and nutritional needs but also to strengthen their fight for liberation from human bondage. Most plantation owners relented and allowed enslaved people to plant their own gardens and produce subsistence crops for their own use as well as for local markets. Early on, a Virginia colonist declared, "There is no master almost [who] will [not] allow his Servant a parcel of clear ground to plant some Tobacco for himself." The pattern persisted into the nineteenth century. One South Carolina slave recalled how his owner limited enslaved people's access to inter-plantation visitations, church-building, and literacy but allotted bondmen and women acreage to till on their own behalf. He gave every one of his plantation families "so much land to plant for dey garden, and den he give em evey Saturday for day time to tend dat garden."[86]

Bondmen and women used these small garden plots to raise corn, peas, squash, and sometimes sweet potatoes. Such garden vegetables supplemented their regular diet of corn and pork. One ex-slave wrote that "every plantation" had gardens, "patches, as they are called . . . in which they plant corn, potatoes, pumpkins, melons, etc. for themselves." Enslaved people not only supplemented their diets with green vegetables but also with "game acquired from hunting, fishing, and "scavenging."[87]

In addition to fighting for their own plots of land and forging their own internal network of medical practitioners, African Americans devised mechanisms for easing the work regimen and protecting their health and well-being as much as possible. Enslaved urban Blacks insisted on contracts that insulated them from some of the most dangerous jobs, especially in the coal and iron industry. In 1825, one owner told an ironmaster that "his bondsman says that working in the furnace is ruinous to his eyes therefore I do not wish him to work there against his will." Similarly, another owner informed an employer about his "man Will"—emphasizing that he did not want Will "to work in the ore or blowing rock as he has been so much injured by it and he is very dissatisfied at it—but he is willing to work at anything that thear is not so much danger." Still another employer consented to let "my boy George . . . work at the blacksmith trade," but added emphatically, "I want you to understand me fully, I do not want him to work at the ore bank."

Most significant, in the long run, however, enslaved and free Blacks gradually developed their own formal churches, fraternal orders, and mutual benefit societies with an eye for serving their health, living conditions, and burial needs as well as their leisure time, cultural, and political pursuits. As early as 1787, in Boston, a group of Blacks formed the Prince Hall Masonic order. The organization soon formed female auxiliaries, established mutual benefit funds, and spread from the urban Northeast to Baltimore, Washington, DC, and Richmond.[88] In 1835, a group of Black ministers reported some thirty-five active Black fraternal societies in Baltimore, each with up to 150 members or more. Nearly a dozen Black women's organizations served the needs of Baltimore's Black community under such names as the Star in the East Association, the Female Ebenezer Association, and the Daughters of Jerusalem.

In some cases, the establishment of early African American labor unions served both mutual benefit and workplace organizing functions. In 1838, Baltimore's Black caulkers formed the Baltimore Caulkers Organization to meet both the mutual benefit and labor needs of Black workers, including the fight against displacement by German and Irish workers from the caulking trade. By 1856, the caulkers continued their labor and mutual benefit work under the rubric of the Baltimore Association of Black Caulkers. In Richmond, "to care for the sick, look after the poor and destitute, and bury their dead," enslaved and free Blacks formed the Poor Saints Fund in 1848 and the United Sons of Love at about the same time. Likewise, the Capital City's Resolute Beneficial Society not only aided the sick and poor in Washington, DC, but also opened a school for Black youth.[89]

In Savannah, Charleston, and New Orleans, African Americans established a variety of mutual benefit organizations to address the health and social welfare needs of free people of color. Although they did not follow their Northern counterparts in setting up chapters of the Prince Hall Masonic orders, these self-help organizations "loaned money to members, cared for orphans and widows, and helped to defray burial expenses of deceased members." In 1790, Charleston's free Black elite founded the exclusive Brown Fellowship Society to serve the needs of light-skinned Black artisans.

The organization devoted the bulk of its time assisting its own members with burial grounds, loans for business development, and aid to children of deceased members who left insufficient estates to secure the welfare of their families. Formed in 1803, the Minor's Moralist Society in Charleston addressed the housing, food, clothing, health, and other social welfare needs of both orphan and "indigent colored children." In 1839, the city's free Black elite spearheaded the formation of the Christian Benevolent Society for the "aid of the sick poor of our free Colored Community in the City, by pecuniary grants, and Judicious Council." Over the next decade and a half, the organization disbursed over $1,200 to some seventy individuals and families.[90]

Through their own myriad efforts to improve their work, housing, and living conditions, the enslaved Black population increased at a rate of about 23 percent from the 1820s through the beginning of the Civil War. Planters repeatedly took credit for this tremendous achievement, claiming "benign" slave labor management policies as the source, but credit belonged to the enslaved people themselves. While their self-activities were insufficient to fundamentally alter their work, health, and living conditions, the cumulative result of their ongoing struggles to improve their lives proved critical to the survival and development of the African American community. Their efforts succeeded against the backdrop of recurring episodes of mob violence, assaults on African American neighborhoods, and a very hostile American colonization movement, designed to relocate free people of color on African soil.

At the same time, during recurring epidemics and health crises, Black people provided indispensable service to the larger white population, despite prevailing racist definitions of sickness, death, and human suffering. In 1793, in the wake of the yellow fever epidemic, nearly half of Philadelphia's white population deserted the city for the countryside. Philadelphia abolitionist and physician Benjamin Rush urged the minister Richard Allen and other African Americans to mobilize Black people to serve their distressed white neighbors as "nurses, gravediggers, and drivers of death carts."[91] Rush also invoked religion to reinforce his notions of African people's biological immunity to yellow fever. Since this disease, by God's will "passes by persons of your color," Rush suggested that Blacks were in turn chosen by God as an instrument of service "to attend the sick."

For their part, Allen and other African Americans took increasing calls for help as both an opportunity for remunerated labor and an opportunity to strike a blow at racism. They would also serve as "defacto medical examiners and notaries, telling city authorities about each day's run of dead and ill patients." Through such efforts, Black Philadelphians hoped to secure a place of equality free of harassment in the city's culture, institutions, and body politic, including access to health care. Following their lifesaving service to the community, however, white residents did little to open the door wider to better health, work, and living conditions for Black citizens. Instead, during the early nineteenth century, Philadelphia's Black community would endure several race riots that left many deaths and injuries and loss of property and homelessness.[92]

Conclusion

The transatlantic slave trade brought some 15 million African people to the New World. North America claimed about a half million of these enslaved Africans. This was only a small fraction of the total number of Africans enslaved in the New World (about 3 percent). Yet, by 1860, the African American population had increased to an estimated 4 million people. A half million of these Black people were free people of color. Their survival defied racist medical science (both physical and mental health professions), violent experiments on African American bodies, and the harsh labor demands of profit-driven slaveholders. Slave owners and former slave owners repeatedly claimed credit for this achievement. Through "benign" management, they argued, enslaved people received sufficient food, clothing, and health care to survive and thrive under the institution of human bondage.

On the contrary, as this chapter shows, African Americans survived the brutal health and life-destroying institution of slavery through the complicated and ongoing interplay of slave owners' self-interest in preserving the health and productivity of the workforce; the rise of a dynamic and aggressive Euro-American medical profession; and, most of all, African Americans' own extraordinary resolve, resistance, and community-building activities. They created their own innovative health care system and forged ways to combat, alleviate, and survive some of the most destructive impacts of enslavement on the health and well-being of Black people. In the years during and following the Civil War and emancipation, as they made the transition from enslaved bondmen and women to citizens in the republic, they would again turn toward their own resources and ingenuity to challenge the persistence of racial and class inequality in the American health care system.

CHAPTER TWO

Emancipation

Introduction

The Civil War and emancipation resulted in the most profound upheaval in the health and health care of African Americans since the nation's founding in the late eighteenth century. War and reconstruction economics and politics disrupted plantation-based medical treatment, including the system that enslaved people had created to treat and cure themselves. With few resources at their disposal, the landless freed people gained only limited access to necessary medical treatment. In the words of O. O. Howard, director of the federal Freedmen's Bureau, "The sudden collapse of the rebellion, making emancipation an actual, universal fact, was like an earthquake. It shook and shattered the whole previously existing social system."[1]

Creation of the federal Freedmen's Bureau in March 1865 and its Medical Division in June slowly addressed the disease and suffering of newly emancipated people, but the government closed its doors in 1872 and turned the health care of emancipated African Americans over to hostile state and local authorities in the South. During the early years of sympathetic Radical Republican regimes, however, these Southern municipalities and states gradually incorporated African Americans into public health services. But the subsequent rise to power of the Democratic Party, the so-called Redeemer segregationist governments, undercut the movement of African Americans into the public health system.[2]

Meanwhile, as postbellum Black people navigated the shifting political regimes on their quest for adequate medical care, they gradually reentered the workforce as sharecroppers, farmhands, and wage-earning laborers in a variety of rural, semirural, urban, and urban industrial jobs. Postbellum labor contracts not only routinely excluded health services for Black workers and their families but also confined Black workers to the most hazardous health- and life-threatening jobs on the bottom rungs of the occupational hierarchy. In addition to offering low wages and few opportunities to move up into higher-paid categories of semiskilled, skilled, and professional work, these jobs exposed African Americans to higher rates of disease, suffering, and death than their white counterparts. The violence and trauma that accompanied the Civil War and Reconstruction upset not only the physical but also the emotional and spiritual well-being of many African Americans, despite the euphoria and celebrations of emancipation and the abolition of slavery.

Similar to their antebellum fight to cure themselves both spiritually and physically, emancipation-era Blacks moved to restore and expand the medical infrastructure that the carnage of war had disrupted and, in many cases, demolished. Rising numbers of African Americans left the plantation community for an uncertain life behind Union lines. In the face of these exceedingly difficult and challenging times, African American health struggles unfolded as part of a larger and more comprehensive fight for full citizenship rights, land, homes, equitable labor contracts, the franchise, and education for themselves and their children. The federal government, philanthropic organizations, and Republican allies of freed people gradually took up what David McBride, eminent historian of Black health care, called "the health equality idea."[3] African Americans and their white allies waged these heroic health care battles within the larger context of severe dislocations in the socioeconomic, epidemiological, and political geography of the postbellum South and nation.[4]

"Biological Crisis," War, and Postbellum Health Care

The Civil War, historian Jim Downs concludes, "produced the largest biological crisis of the nineteenth century," claiming "more soldiers' lives" and resulting in "more casualties than battle or warfare." The war also wreaked "havoc on the population of the newly freed."[5]

As the Civil War got underway, African Americans escaped from Southern plantations in rising numbers. They made their way to widely dispersed Union encampments as the war picked up steam and federal forces penetrated the slaveholding South. US military and government officials soon established "contraband camps" to house the massive numbers of fugitives who moved into Union lines. These "contraband" of war were swiftly put to work on behalf of the Union Army. Men constructed fortifications, tended livestock, and carried out numerous manual labor tasks associated with military service, while women cooked, washed clothes, and served as nurses for the injured and sick. Black women like Harriet Tubman, Sojourner Truth, and Susie King Taylor provided yeoman nursing services to the US military forces during the Civil War. Some of the men were eventually recruited into the Union Army as soldiers.[6]

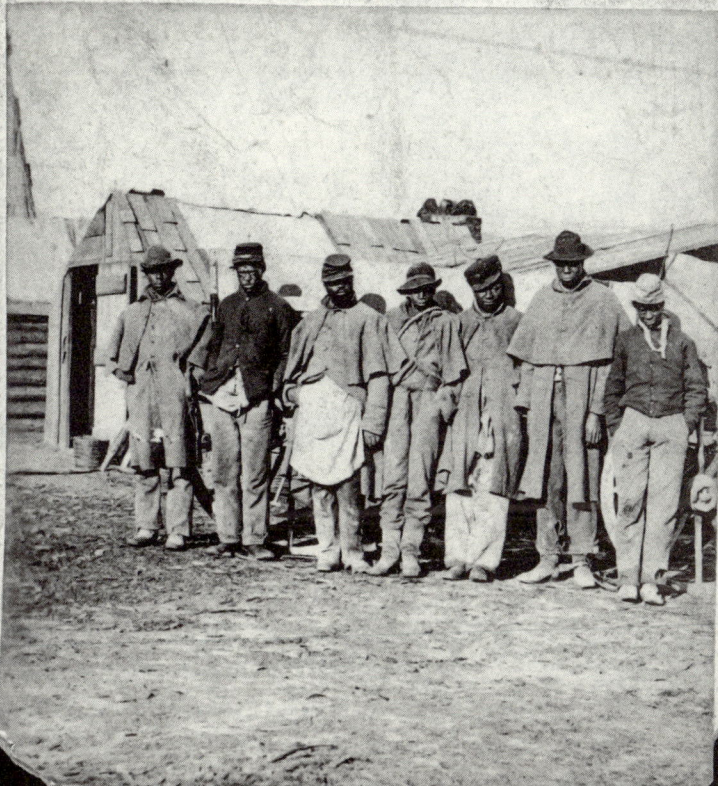

Colored (Union) Army teamsters, Cobb Hill, Va. (1864). Photographer, John C. Taylor, stereograph. Library of Congress, Prints and Photographs Division.

War, Disease, and New Health Challenges

African American men like Martin Delany gained renown for their medical services to Union troops during the Civil War, but Black soldiers occupied a "second class status" that took a huge toll on their health and well-being. As historian Margaret Humphreys notes, "Medical care for black soldiers was inadequate, and their hospitals were poorly supplied." Furthermore, to paraphrase Humphreys, African Americans were not only "frequently ill" but

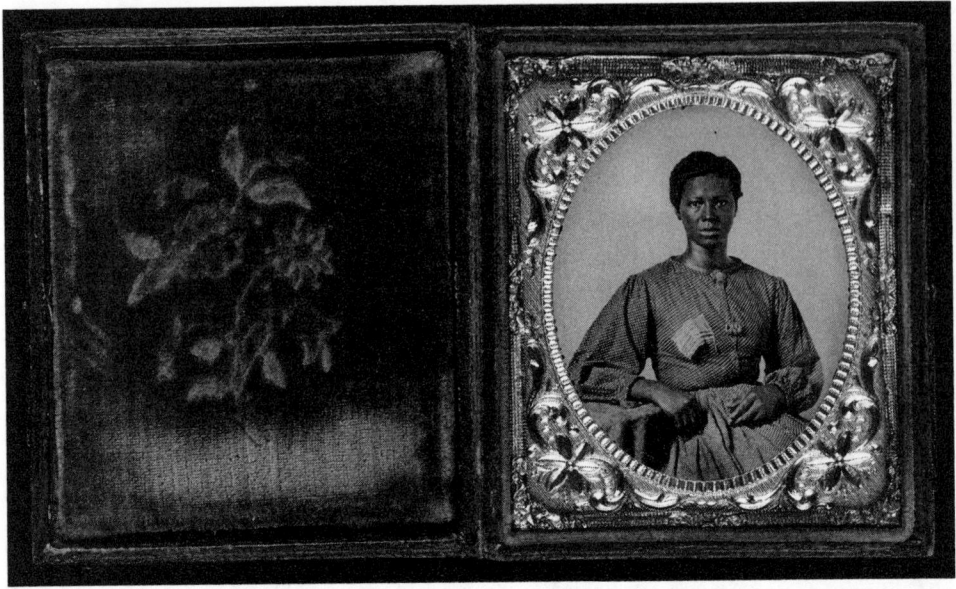

Washerwoman for the Union Army, Richmond, Virginia (1862–65). Photographer unknown. National Museum of American History, Division of Work and Industry, Smithsonian Institution.

also "frequently ill served" by the medical profession. The ideology of general Black biological inferiority seemingly migrated with the transition from slavery to freedom. When questioned about his maltreatment of Black troops under his care, one negligent surgeon retorted that "it was useless to doctor a sick negro, for he was sure to die, do what you would."[7]

Whereas disease took down the majority of Black and white soldiers during the Civil War, military combat claimed the lives of more white than Black soldiers. An estimated 4.5 percent of white soldiers died in battle compared to 1.8 percent for African Americans. Conversely, however, about 13.5 percent of white men lost their lives during wartime service in contrast to 18.5 percent for Black men, a product of the disproportionately higher mortality rate of Black soldiers suffering from various diseases. Disease by disease, African American soldiers endured higher mortality rates than their white counterparts. Their mortality rate for pneumonia was four times greater than their white counterparts; ten times higher for scurvy; three times higher for tuberculosis; and five times higher for smallpox.

Even for malaria (a disease for which African Americans were widely acknowledged as particularly immune compared to whites), the Black mortality rate was about three times more fatal for Black than white soldiers.[8] Moreover, fugitives not only brought into Union lines the damage done to their bodies by plantation slavery but also the additional wounds inflicted by the hazards of escape during the socioeconomic and political upheavals of war. Ira Russell, a sympathetic Massachusetts army physician, later described how large numbers of fugitives arrived in the war zones of St. Louis, Missouri, and the East Coast "in feeble health, with impaired constitutions, broken down by exposure and privation while escaping from their masters, or from crowding in contraband camps [elsewhere] and bad and insufficient diet."[9]

Large numbers of Blacks suffered and died because of poor health care, disease, and epidemics during the early emancipation years following the war. Unsanitary conditions within and beyond military encampments; inadequate food, clothing, and shelter; and the government's forced migration of freed people and their families from one military installation to another—all repeatedly exposed them and their families to widespread disease and suffering. In his pioneering historical synthesis of Black health care, medical historian Herbert M. Morais illuminated the predicament of emancipated people. They were emancipated from the old slave quarters that once provided them "shelter and a modicum of health care." Now they were literally "turned loose, ill-clad, hungry and destitute, waiting and ever hoping" for a better life in tumultuous times. Some newly freed people received "no medical care at all," and "disease and death ran rampant through black populations." To cite one example, at Promised Land, a small rural Black community founded in 1870 about midway between Charleston and Atlanta, residents scattered, many becoming homeless after a promise of land in exchange for their labor collapsed. They had cleared many acres of cotton-producing land in accord with the landowner Old Samuel Marshall's promise: "If you clean two acres you get two acres; if you clean ten acres you get ten acres."[10]

At war's end, one unknown, improperly clothed, and neglected Black youth symbolized the human toll of the Civil War on the health and well-being of newly emancipated people. The child endured freezing winter temperatures, high winds, frostbite, and the likely amputation of his frozen feet. He and his five siblings also lost their mother during the family's forced move from Chattanooga to Nashville and then back to Chattanooga. An estimated one-quarter to one-third of the formerly enslaved population died in some Southern communities during the first years after freedom. According to medical historians W. Michael Byrd and Linda Clayton, the reconstruction and post-reconstruction years were traumatic for former slaves as "new waves of epidemics [including excessively high rates of tuberculosis], poor health, sickness and death swept through the postwar South."[11]

Established in the US War Department in the spring of 1865, the Freedmen's Bureau helped to alleviate the suffering of many newly emancipated people with mixed results. Before its termination in 1872, the bureau had established over forty hospitals and almshouses, and employed over a hundred doctors and "countless" nurses, stewards, and aides to provide medical services to freed people.[12] Under the leadership of Dr. Robert Reyburn, an Irish-born white surgeon, the Freedmen's Bureau transformed one contraband camp called "Camp Barker" into the Freedmen's Hospital and Asylum, which later became the teaching hospital for Howard University's medical school. No more than 140 physicians were responsible for serving some 1.1 million people who populated the government-sponsored camps for refugees. Moreover, some of the white physicians openly resisted providing services to the legions of freed people seeking medical attention. One physician referred to the emancipated people as "animals" in the company of the camp's relief workers.[13]

Other physicians, health officials, and the popular press used the postbellum health crisis to challenge the wisdom of emancipation itself. When one newly freed Alabama woman gave birth to her child on the ground and then climbed into a dump cart to recover, "hogs came along and ate her infant." Pro-confederate newspapers declared that "such a thing would never have occurred under slavery." Furthermore, according to the *Montgomery Daily Ledger*, as slaves, Black people were healthier people. They "could be up early and late, labor hard, expose themselves in all kinds of weather and seldom complain or take to their beds. Now . . . the least exposure throws them."[14] One planter in Alabama's Lowndes County explained to his former bondmen and women: "Formerly, you were my slaves; you worked for me, and I provided for you [including medical care]. . . . But now all that is changed. Being free men, you assume the responsibilities of free men. You sell me your labor, I pay you money, and with that money you provide for yourselves." A Virginian stated simply: "I do not like the negro as well free as I did as a slave. . . . Then, I was always thinking of how I could fix him comfortably. Now, I find myself driving a hard bargain with him for wages."[15]

The postbellum Southern medical profession also intensified its belief that freedom and not slavery and its destructive aftermath underlay the rise in mental illness among newly emancipated people. Unlike the years of enslavement, however, when few institutions acknowledged or admitted disabled or mentally ill African Americans, except in the case of the small but growing free Black population, particularly in the North, postbellum institutions for the mentally ill not only admitted rising numbers of Black people as patients but depended on their labor to help reconstruct and sustain the life of the institution at a time when resources were few and declining for all disabled and mentally challenged people, Black and white. While whites would continue to receive where possible rehabilitative and restorative services aimed at returning them to their families and communities, African Americans would receive admittance with an eye on their capacity to earn their own keep, provide unpaid labor on the institution's agricultural land, and enrich the institution's white professional staff. Although the modern psychiatric concept of "stress" would only gain currency during the twentieth century, it certainly affected the lives of countless African Americans during the upheaval of the war and early postwar years.[16]

In the fall of 1865, the federal government set up a Freedmen's Bureau unit in Milledgeville, Georgia, near the state's Lunatic, Idiot, and Epileptic Asylum. Initially, when bureau officials sought the admission of Black patients at the facility, the asylum's administrator emphatically rejected the admission of African Americans. At about the same time, a special Georgia state legislative committee that was established to study the issue concluded, in the language of the prewar years, that Georgia and by implication the entire South would likely see "insanity in the negro much more common under the new dispensation [meaning freedom] than it was under the old code" of slavery. Still, the Milledgeville institution only opened its doors to Blacks following mounting federal pressure from Freedmen's Bureau officials. Between August and December 1867, the first group of African Americans gained admission to the facility. Among a total of seventy-four patients admitted during the period, there were forty-four African Americans (thirty women and fourteen men), nearly half arriving from Freedmen's hospitals across the state of Georgia.[17]

Rather than integrating Blacks into the existing architecture of the asylum, the state and psychiatry professionals constructed a new "Colored Building" to house the freed men and women. With the arrival of rising numbers of Black patients, medical and state authorities replaced an earlier emphasis on "moral therapy" in the treatment of white patients with a new racialized labor, productivity, and profit-oriented regime. The work potential of newly freed men and women took center stage in their treatment protocol. Instead of measuring success in the number of people restored to mental health and returned to their families and communities, the institution expanded its agricultural production and gauged its success by the mounting profits of its "pigs and cows in the farm and garden section," all thanks to the unpaid labor of patients deemed mentally ill and disabled. As popular mental health scholar Mab Segrest persuasively argues, the state's

Lunatic, Idiot, and Epileptic Asylum placed Georgia "at the epicenter of race and psychiatry into the twentieth century."[18]

Race, Inequality, and the Medical Profession

The medical profession nonetheless gradually changed some of its earlier class and racial biases against poor and working-class Blacks and whites. During the 1880s, scientists and medical professionals isolated the principal organisms responsible for tuberculosis, diphtheria, cholera, and typhoid. Over the next decade, medical researchers devised successful laboratory tests for detecting these maladies and prescribing cures. As historical sociologist Paul Starr notes, chemical and bacteriological tests for disease rapidly unfolded as the twentieth century got underway. A substantial segment of the medical profession gradually backed away from "moral interpretations" of disease as a product of what they had earlier described as the debilitating lifestyles of the poor.[19]

Despite gradual shifts in medical ideas and practices, white supremacist interpretations of disease persisted and even intensified with the rise of the Jim Crow order. In some cases, the adoption of new technology like the spirometer, an instrument for measuring the lung capacity of human beings, reinforced the racialization of medical science. Benjamin Gould, a researcher for the US Sanitary Commission, used the spirometer to produce a body of research showing marked differences in the lung capacity of Black and white soldiers. According to Gould, "full blooded" African American men (an exceedingly problematic characterization since few African Americans could be considered "full blooded" Negro) "blew ten to twenty cubic inches of air less than their white comrades." In her study of Black Civil War soldiers, historian Margaret Humphreys underscored how the differential lung capacity of Blacks and whites might have influenced how well they could fight off diseases like pneumonia. However, in her groundbreaking research on the instrument, historian Lundy Braun concludes that "race became a key organizing principle of spirometry in *dialogue with* other categories of difference—including occupation, social class, gender, and disability— whose cultural salience changed over time and place."[20]

The medical profession and most white Americans clung to the idea of African American biological inferiority and hence their greater susceptibility than whites to all sorts of contagious diseases, including diphtheria, syphilis, typhus, and tuberculosis (TB), to name a few. In the hands of white supremacist medical professionals, such new medical technology like the spirometer confirmed their belief in innate differences between Blacks and whites and the inferiority of Black bodies in comparison. Overall, according to David McBride, mainstream American society as well as the medical profession "viewed black Americans more as a source of contagion than as fellow victims" confronting debilitating diseases like TB.[21]

Frederick L. Hoffman, the German-born chief statistician for the Prudential Life Insurance Company, emerged as the most prominent proponent of the new scientific racism. Based on an assessment of countless medical reports and quantitative health insurance documents, Hoffman predicted the gradual extinction of the Black race. He also convinced the nation's leading insurance companies to treat African Americans, given their imminent mortality, as "uninsurable." Hoffman's influential study on *Race Traits and Tendencies of the American Negro* (1896) became a popular text for medical school classes on race and disease. An early postbellum study by E. W. Gilliam ("The African American in the United States," published in 1883 in the *Popular Science Monthly*) persuasively suggested that Black population growth "was outstripping that of Whites."[22]

When confronted with Gilliam's evidence, Hoffman quickly reassured the white supremacist scientific and medical community that, "in spite of their fecundity . . . in the struggle for race supremacy the black race is not holding its own; and eventual extinction was inevitable." Hoffman further concluded that inherent "racial inferiority" of Black people ensured that they would perennially suffer higher death rates than whites, "even under the same conditions." In a professional medical journal, another white medical supremacist, Charles S. Bacon, offered an even more extreme and impatient read of the evidence. Bacon said that "he did not doubt the 'eventual elimination' of blacks in the United States. However, since the latest census data indicated that the 'race is not doomed . . . in the immediate future," he emphatically suggested "helping along the process of extinction," implying support for even greater barriers on African American access to life-sustaining medical care.[23]

Other influential advocates of the new racism in the medical profession included Robert Shufeldt and a host of physicians and public health officials in the South. The Georgian Daniel D. Quillian; the Mississippian H. M. Folkes; and the Virginian Thomas W. Murrell, all enthusiastically endorsed the Englishman Herbert Spencer's translation of Charles Darwin's "evolutionary theory" into a nearly ironclad racist framework for understanding health and human history. Daniel D. Quillian of Athens, Georgia, in an essay titled "Race Peculiarities of the Prevalence of Syphilis in Negroes" (1906), concluded that people of African descent were "natives of tropical and semitropical climates" where "sexual instincts" had developed to an extraordinary extent. When combined with African Americans' presumed "lax morals and indifference to virtue," Quillian argued that African people are thus "more prone to venereal disease than the white race."

Furthermore, Quillian reported, "Virtue in the negro race is like angels' visits—few and far between. In a practice of sixteen years in the South I have never examined a virgin over fourteen years of age." Likewise, in his studies on "The Negro as a Health Problem" and "Syphilis and the American Negro: A Medico-Sociologic Study," physician T. W. Murrell of Richmond, Virginia, reinforced the racist interpretation of syphilis and other diseases among Blacks during the first generation following emancipation. Murrell strongly accented his belief that freedom itself had opened the door for the presumed inherent depravity of the Black race to gain expression. In a vicious medical diatribe against Black people, he said, African Americans were now "absolutely free to gratify his every sexual impulse; to be infested with every loathsome disease and infect his ready and willing companion—and he did it—he did it all. The result is the negro of 1909, the negro of today." Murrell further declared, "It is my honest belief that another fifty years will find an unsyphilitic negro a freak."[24]

Murrell, Quillian, Hoffman, and legions of professional and popular writers like them claimed a fundamental connection between "phenotypical race traits" (particularly skin color) and all aspects of the human condition, including mental illness, crime, criminality, and even presumably "low levels of intelligence" among people of African descent. Above all, these writers expressed an abiding belief in the eventual obliteration of the Black race. Historian John S. Haller, in his classic study of white supremacist thought, underscored the new racial consensus on the fate of Black people. Despite the immense complexity of the issue and "the reservations of many," Haller said, "the belief in the Negro's extinction became one of the most pervasive ideas in American medical and anthropological thought during the late nineteenth century. It was a fitting culmination to the [long held] concept of racial inferiority in American life."[25]

Reinforcing the Groundwork for Medical Jim Crow

Across the late nineteenth and early twentieth century, the nation's medical establishment withheld the benefits of cutting-edge medical treatment from African Americans. Before the Civil War, for example, the medical profession had largely contained smallpox through an effective system of quarantines and vaccinations. Yet, between 1862 and 1868, when a smallpox epidemic broke out across the South and took the lives of thousands of African Americans, the Medical Division of the Freedmen's Bureau failed to institute effective measures to contain the virus among formerly enslaved people. Instead, bureau officials believed that the high mortality rate of Blacks from the disease confirmed their "inferiority" as a people and was a sure sign of the impending "extinction of the black race."[26] Hence, leaders of the Medical Division "did not provide Bureau physicians . . . with adequate money and resources" to meet the health challenges of emancipated people.[27] Moreover, as TB spread across the country and took Black lives at three times the rate of their white counterparts during the 1880s, 1890s, and beyond, racist portraits of the disease prevailed. When it became clear that TB claimed rising numbers of whites as well as Blacks, the medical profession tended to portray white TB sufferers as "victims," while treating Blacks, especially Black women household workers, as "perpetrators" or "carriers" of the disease.[28]

In Atlanta, the anti-TB movement publicized the case of Minnie Freeman, a young Black washerwoman and TB victim. Freeman lived and worked in close proximity to "one of the most pretentious and popular residence streets in the whole city of Atlanta." She presumably represented "the most dangerous case on the records of the tuberculosis clinic" and "threw off the germs of a terrible disease—enough to infect the whole city." Regularly referred to as the "great white plague," symptoms of the disease included "wasting away, coughing, spitting, and weakening" of the body. Fear of Blacks spreading this disease also presumably represented an opportunity for white Atlantans to close their own class gap and fight the Black "scourge." As the *Atlanta Constitution* concluded, in addition to the washerwoman, Black nurses, cooks, chauffeurs, butlers, and laborers of all sorts would "come from within the pale" and "bring the bacilli from the segregated district into the homes of the poor and rich white Atlantans . . . and scatter disease."[29]

Limitations on African American access to needed health care were closely related to the increasing class as well as racial stratification of the American health system. The expanding use of surgery to address acute illnesses during the late nineteenth and early twentieth century gradually transformed the hospital from a place for the long-term care of poor and "indigent patients," for whom hospital stays lasted as much as a month or more, to a place of much shorter stays for poor people with chronic ailments of various sorts. Hospitals gave increasing attention to fee-paying white elite patients requiring expensive surgeries and longer-term care. At the Massachusetts General

Hospital in Boston, hospital stays for poor patients dropped below four weeks for the first time in 1886. A decade later, average stays at the facility continued to drop to just days rather than weeks.[30]

As class restrictions limited the white poor's access to health care, they pushed African American patients even further down the scale. In 1906, for example, in Washington, DC, the Board of Charities reported that government funding had created too many small hospitals "for acute medical and surgical services" for the elite and "utterly failed" to provide for the care of "chronic, convalescent, tubercular, inebriate, and generally undesirable cases." The city reported only one hospital under its "direct control," and it was "constantly overcrowded with general chronic cases, which are not desired and which will not be received by institutions not under the immediate control of the city." As Starr notes, "This pattern became a standard feature of American medicine—a highly developed private sector for acute treatment and an underdeveloped public sector for chronic care. Private hospitals for acute illness would be running well below capacity, while overcrowded public institutions were teeming with the victims of tuberculosis, alcoholism, mental disorder, and other diseases of social disorganization."[31]

Unequal sharecropping agreements and wage labor contracts deepened the health crisis confronting Black people. Authorities focused almost exclusively on identifying "able bodied" men and "their ability to work" in the reconfigured free labor Southern workforce. They downplayed the employment and health requirements of Black women and their children.[32] During the antebellum years, Black women and children were employed in remunerative work. But postbellum federal officials redefined women and children as dependents of Black men and severely circumscribed their access to viable paid work. Hence, freed women and children figured prominently among people defined as "destitute" and requiring public and charitable relief. According to Freedmen's Bureau records, nearly 5,300 freed women needed relief in Tennessee compared to 1,000 freed men. Similarly, in Virginia, an estimated 8,900 freed women received public rations compared to 3,000 freed men.[33]

As freed people navigated the depths of medical inequality, scientific racism, and the horrors of the early postbellum disease environment, federal military authorities, the Freedmen's Bureau, and state and local governments underwrote a new combined sharecropping, wage, and carceral labor system. Postbellum governments in the South established stringent public policies to force able-bodied Black men into the workforce on exceedingly unequal terms with their employers.

Agricultural Labor and New Industrial Health Hazards

At the core of this new labor system were a series of legislative measures, the "Black Codes," vagrancy laws that made unemployment (even temporary unemployment) a criminal offense. At the same time, a plethora of supplemental anti-enticement laws made it a crime for an employer to hire a worker still under contract with another employer. Labor contracts ordinarily placed medical costs on the shoulders of the sharecropper. Where such landowners did take responsibility for health care, they still passed the costs on to Black workers and their families. In June 1865, for example, A. J. Donelson, a former slave owner signed a contract with his sharecroppers, including attending to the sick at a cost of "twenty-five cents for each dose of medicine, and one dollar for every time he may be called to prescribe."[34] Southern landowning elites believed that their own class interests and the interests of the South required that they command African American labor "completely, or the production of the cotton crop must be abandoned."[35]

Violence, Health, and the Politics of Coerced Labor

Reminiscent of slave ownership, postbellum landowners regularly extolled the whip as the great secret of their economic success as cotton growers before the Civil War, and they vowed to continue the practice in managing their free Black workforce. The ubiquitous use of violence repeatedly blurred distinctions in the labor experiences of Black people across municipal, county, and state boundaries. A Mississippi planter declared his resolve to "go right on like we always did . . . and I pole 'em if they don't do right." The same planter placed his right to employ the whip in his labor contract with Black workers. He gleefully reported, "I put it into the contract that I was to whoop 'em when I pleased."[36] In 1905, one Georgia cotton sharecropping hand recalled how he had been whipped as a young man during the 1880s for daring to seek employment on another sharecropping place. The landowner employed local law enforcement officers to locate and return him to the place. As he recalled, "That night he made me strip off my clothing down to my waist, ordered his foreman to give me thirty lashes with a buggy whip across my bare back, and stood by until it was done. After that experience, the Captain made me stay on his place night and day."[37]

The rise of Radical Republican governments eased somewhat the harshest features of early postbellum health care, race, and labor relations. In state after state during the late 1860s and early 1870s, radical legislators initiated the gradual movement of African Americans into the Southern health care system, including public hospitals in Richmond, Virginia, and Montgomery, Alabama, mostly on a segregated basis.[38] Before African Americans could secure an equitable economic footing and improve their access to better work, health, and living conditions under radical political regimes, however, the Democratic Party regained control of state and local governments. Calling themselves "redeemers" of Southern society, Southern Democrats strengthened the hand of the landowners and weakened the bargaining position of Black workers.[39]

New constraints on the livelihood of Black workers and their families included "sunset" and "fence" laws. Since sharecropping agreements mandated labor from "dawn to dusk," there was little time for African Americans to market the produce of their gardens except at night. "Sunset laws" prohibited farm tenants from selling their produce "after dark" and deprived rural Blacks of an important part of their livelihood. The new "fence laws" cut even deeper into the health and well-being of tenant farmers and sharecroppers. In the past, Southern law protected the right of farmers to allow their livestock "to roam and feed upon any unfenced land." Fence laws removed this source of livelihood for scores of Black agricultural workers and farm families. These regulations required farmers to raise cattle and hogs in "enclosed pastures, which many sharecroppers and tenant farmers did not have." At the same time, other legal restrictions curtailed hunting, fishing, foraging, and squatting on vacant, "unfenced land" and effectively "cut off the lifeline of many rural black households."[40]

By 1900, nearly 80 percent of Blacks in the South worked as share or cash tenants on land owned by whites. In the meantime, the boll weevil crossed the Mexican border into the southwestern United States during the 1890s. It traveled quickly eastward, passing the Mississippi River by 1910. As Swedish scholar Gunnar Myrdal stated in his massive survey of African American life, "One state after another in the Old South was hit. The destruction was terrible." The Alabama sharecropper and later landowner Ned Cobb (also known as Nate Shaw) later recalled the devastation on his place, declaring that "all God's dangers aint a white man."[41] In Georgia and South Carolina, many landowners "permanently abandoned" their plantations and farms as the boll weevil devastated the cotton crop.[42]

When landowners abandoned the land and discontinued cotton cultivation, African American workers faced displacement and sometimes eviction from the land as sharecroppers and tenants. Their quest for employment and new homes revealed how both unemployment and exploitative labor arrangements made them especially vulnerable to disease, sickness, and poor health. As early as 1880, a US Census Bureau report described rural Black life as "destitute . . . many are in worse condition than they were during slavery." In 1910, a Northern minister visited the South and declared that "the wretchedness is pathetic and the poverty colossal."[43]

As suggested by the ravages of the boll weevil, the sharecropping system not only entailed exploitative work and labor relations but also destructive environmental conditions that undermined the health and well-being of Blacks and whites. Nonetheless, racially discriminatory social policies and practices reinforced the disproportionate impact of these conditions on the lives of Black workers and their families. When the so-called Redeemers gained control of state and local governments in the South, some authorities closed public hospitals and eliminated systems of outdoor relief for the poor, including health care. They often claimed that radicals had used these services as a means of securing the Black vote.[44]

In 1875, for instance, when Democrats in Montgomery, Alabama, seized control of city government, the new mayor promptly "closed the city hospital" as part of his severe retrenchment program. Similarly, the state legislature shuttered the Freemen's Hospital, located near Talladega. At about the same time, Nashville Redeemers abolished the city's system of outdoor relief, pointedly accusing the Republican mayor of "using poor relief as a device to attract Negro voters to his party." For its part, Atlanta eliminated the office of "Warden of the poor." It transferred the duty of dispensing outdoor relief to the police department "to assure that applicants," particularly poor Blacks, received close scrutiny.[45]

Redeemers were also responsible for reinforcing and extending patterns of racial violence against the first generation of free people well into the twentieth century. Southern and Northern urbanites backed up their opposition to Black settlement by violence. As lynchings engulfed Blacks in the countryside, urban whites adopted the race riot as their principal form of mob violence. Destructive race riots broke out in New Orleans and Memphis in 1866; Philadelphia in 1871; Danville, Virginia, in 1883; Wilmington, North Carolina, in 1898; New York in 1900; Atlanta in 1906; and Springfield, Illinois, in 1904 and 1908. White mobs entered Black communities, destroyed property, and beat, killed, and injured scores of people, forcing many to flee for their lives. Invariably, local police joined the mobs in their attacks, while other officials, including mayors and governors, aided and abetted the violence by their overt actions or inaction as public servants responsible for insuring public safety. Moreover, some of the violence involved outright lynchings. In Nashville, for example, brutal lynchings of Blacks occurred in 1872, 1875, 1877, and 1890.

Following the downfall of Radical Reconstruction, lynchings of African Americans escalated. This brutal form of mob law averaged 100 per year during the 1880s and 1890s, peaking at 161 in 1892. The leading authority on lynching statistics, the Tuskegee Institute's annual *Negro Year Book*, recorded that lynchings reached 3,130 between 1882 and 1901; nearly 2,000 were Blacks, including 40 Black women out of a total of 63 women victims. Although the number of recorded lynchings gradually declined by 1910, the brutality of such atrocities intensified. Lynchers burned, tortured, and dismembered their Black victims, while public officials and law enforcement officers aided and abetted the process and helped to cement white bonds of community at African Americans' expense, as suggested by the photo of a Paris, Texas, lynching.

Lynchings and mob attacks on Black communities and neighborhoods reinforced racial disparities in the US medical system. Scholars are only now beginning to give appropriate attention to the ongoing impact of racial violence on the mental as well as the physical health of Black people.[46] But these violent assaults on the African American population included state violence as well as white citizen attacks. In 1889, for example, in Leflore County, Mississippi, when Black farmers sought to organize a Black farmer's alliance to control the price of their crops, grown at great sacrifice by the sweat of their brow, a white citizen mob attacked the community. But their assault was turned back by massive numbers of armed Black men determined to defend themselves, their families, and their communities against mob violence. When the mobs encountered stiff and successful resistance, they called for help from local and state law enforcement agents. In this case, as the white mob retreated in the face of the armed Black community, the Mississippi National Guardsmen took charge of murdering from 30 to 100 Black people.[47]

Along with the impact of public policies and mob rule on the health and well-being of Black communities, poor housing and living conditions also exacerbated the health challenges confronting postbellum and Jim Crow era Black communities. African Americans inherited much of their housing stock from the antebellum slave regime. Most were small, one-room wooden houses with dirt floors and fireplaces as the only source of heat and light. Few of these structures had windows with glass panes or even wooden shutters. Moreover, cracks in the walls and holes in the ceilings exposed freed men, women, and their children to the rain, wind, and insects. As agricultural historian Gilbert C. Fite makes clear, the wooden shutters were left open during the summer months "to admit air and light." In addition to open shutters, holes in the walls, roofs, and floors also let in flies, mosquitoes, and other insects, including snakes. In 1895, in a rural shack near Tuskegee, Alabama, one Black woman reported that snakes sometimes crawled into her abode, but she "just bresh 'em out." At Promised Land and elsewhere across the rural South, many of the wooden houses with fireplaces and wood stove "burned to the ground, leaving families homeless."[48]

Born in Randolph County, Alabama, during the 1870s, William Henry Holtzclaw, a Tuskegee graduate and founder of a vocational institute for Black youth, later recalled growing up in a small "fourteen-by sixteen-foot windowless split-pine cabin" structure that had previously housed enslaved Blacks on the large plantation. Holtzclaw not only remembered how he and his family were inadequately sheltered, but also how they were inadequately clothed and fed: "Dressed in simple, one-piece shifts made out of burlap sacks, the children went barefoot year round and began work at an early age," he said. "Food was so scarce. I was hungry all the time. . . . We were emaciated, underfed little creatures."[49]

Prelude to the Urban Industrial Age

Although sharecropping emerged as the dominant labor system in the postbellum cotton South and shaped patterns of migration, work, housing, and living conditions across the nation, it was by no means universal.[50] As in the prewar years, tobacco, sugar, and rice followed different patterns of production and generated different forms of work, housing, health, and living conditions. In Virginia and North Carolina, tobacco growers preferred wage labor and offered few opportunities for Blacks to gain their own plots of land or work on shares.[51] Northern capital poured into the Louisiana sugar industry. Compared to the antebellum sugar regime, however, newly freed Black workers curbed the labor intensity of sugar production and eased the deleterious impact of such work on their health. They placed a high priority on their own plots and used harvest time to bargain for higher wages and better work and living conditions. Consequently, the life expectancy of postbellum sugar workers gradually increased over the short lifespan of their enslaved counterparts.[52]

In the postbellum rice fields, landownership and independent production allowed ex-slaves to shape the terms of their labor, even more so than sugar workers. They discouraged outside capitalist investments in the area and kept rice production relatively low. As one South Carolina ex-slave recalled, bondage provided "no rest, Massa all work, all de time . . . no rest, no re-pose." Freedom on the other hand offered a "chance for [a] little comfort."[53] In the Georgetown rice-growing region of the state, women dramatically re-duced their full-time work in the fields from nearly 70 percent in 1866 to 34 percent in 1868.[54]

Rooted partly in their antebellum industrial work experiences and the de-teriorating conditions of agriculture in the South, postbellum Black work-ers moved into rural and urban industrial jobs in rising numbers. By the onset of World War I, African Americans made up an estimated one-third to a ma-jority of all coal miners in West Virginia and the Birmingham district of Alabama. Across the so-called urban industrial New South, they also helped to lay miles of railroad tracks that opened up access to rich veins of iron ore, coal, phosphate, and forest lands for the lumber industry. In parts of Virginia, West Virginia, and Ohio, for example, Black workers helped to build the Chesapeake and Ohio, the Norfolk and Western, and the Virginian railroads, before entering the coal mines as coal loaders in large numbers.[55]

Each category of industrial work took its own special toll on the health and livelihood of Black workers and their families. Between 1898 and 1907, an estimated one out of every 230 railroad "switchtenders" died every year, "as did one out of every 131 railway trainmen," not to mention the injuries and deaths of the legions of general laborers who prepared railroad beds and laid thousands of miles of track across the country. Some four-fifths of Black workers "endured the South's extreme heat maintaining roadbeds and lay-ing track." In South Carolina, some Black workers moved from the rice fields into the phosphate pits of Charleston, as the city's phosphate industry de-veloped and expanded after 1867. A predominantly Black labor force dug rock from land-based pits as well as collected rock from river beds by dredges. Black laborers also transported the rock to railroad lines so it could then be shipped to mills, where it was crushed into fine powder, treated with acid, and transformed into fertilizer. Phosphate mill operations added to wide-spread respiratory ailments that afflicted large numbers of Black industrial workers.[56]

In the bituminous coal industry, Black and white miners contracted black lung disease, then commonly referred to as "miners' asthma." Still, racial dis-crimination in the assignment of underground workplaces often relegated Black workers to areas with lots of water, rock, and low coal seams, requir-ing them to load coal on their knees more often than their white counter-parts. Lung disease was a slow killer of miners, caused by the repeated inhalation of coal dust, while mine explosions were the most dramatic and publicized cause of miners' deaths. Between 1905 and 1909, the US coal industry reported eighty-five major coal mine disasters that took the lives of over 2,600 miners. The deadliest explosions took place in West Virginia and Pennsylvania. By 1913, the United States counted an estimated "25,000 industrial fatalities and 700,000 injuries involving a disability of more than four weeks among 38 million employed men and women." But day-to-day roof and coal falls accounted for the largest and most consistent cause of death among miners. There was also a special emotional toll that coal mining took on the health of Black families. In an interview on their lives in the southern West Virginia coalfields, one Black miner and his wife later recalled how fear was a prominent part of their lives in the coal town: "That fear was always there all the time, because . . . you may see [each other] in the morning and never [see each other] any more in the flesh."[57]

Iron, steel, and lumber companies also employed Black workers in the most dangerous, life-threatening jobs. In the steel mills of Birmingham, "top fillers" worked atop the furnaces, where "some eighty-feet above ground, they shoveled iron ore into the hopper while risking death from asphyxiation, explosions, and falls." By the early twentieth century, an estimated one in five Black industrial worker labored in the lumber industry, considered "one of the most dangerous industries in early twentieth-century American manufacturing." In logging operations and in sawmills, "dangers lurked everywhere, from bursting saws to falling timbers."[58]

Southern states also erected a new prison system that undermined the health and well-being of Black families by ensnaring an escalating number of Black workers, including the principal breadwinners, in a system of forced labor reminiscent of their experiences as enslaved workers. However, in order to sidestep responsibility for the cost of housing, medical care, and supervision of a huge Black convict population, Georgia, Mississippi, and Alabama, among other states, established a "convict leasing system" that allowed prison authorities to lease Black prisoners to a variety of private employers at huge profit to the state.[59] Contemporary descriptions of the holding areas for convict laborers repeatedly describe such facilities as "little more than cow sheds, horse stables, or hog pens." Disease, suffering, and death were extensive. One ex-convict recalled that few prisoners died during his last ten years in a Georgia "peon camp," but "a great many came away maimed and bruised and, in some cases, disabled for life."[60]

Owners of cotton plantations, lumber mills, coal mines, and railroads hired rising numbers of incarcerated Black men and, to some extent, Black women. Convict labor camps and chain gangs proliferated. Black prisoners labored from sun up to sun down under armed guards, vicious prison dogs, and the whip.[61] Some of the camps employed new and more fiendish ways to punish the men. "A favorite way of whipping a man was to strap him down to a log, flat on his back, and spank him fifty or sixty times on his bare feet with a shingle or a huge piece of plank. When the man would get up with sore and blistered feet and an aching body, if he could not then keep up with other men at work he would be strapped to the log again, this time face downward, and would be lashed with a buggy trace on his bare back." One ex-convict later remembered a Georgia convict camp as "hell itself!"[62]

As suggested by the employment of convict laborers by large numbers of privately owned plantations, railroads, mines, and mills, the line between free wage earners and unfree convict workers blurred considerably. Both rural and urban industrial Black workers, incarcerated and unincarcerated, inhabited the poorest, most segregated, and least healthy environments. In the urban South, most poor and working-class Blacks occupied basic single frame "shotgun houses" and, in some cases, "double shotgun" houses in low-amenity areas of the city.[63] During the 1880s, the Charleston Board of Health described a Black neighborhood in the northeastern part of the city as a "dangerous and unhealthy region." During heavy rains, the area flooded and left pools of stagnant water under houses in the area, which city health officials referred to as "breeding ground for infectious diseases" in the community.

In Florida, following Miami's incorporation as a city in 1896, real estate discrimination confined most of the city's Black population to an area called "Colored Town." Most homes lined unpaved streets, lacked electricity and indoor plumbing, and regularly suffered damage from "heavy rains, winds, and fire."[64] On the eve of World War I, one contemporary study of Birmingham, Alabama, described Black neighborhoods in the city as "nests of infection" for a broad range of diseases, including tuberculosis, typhoid, and cholera. Municipal zoning laws and discriminatory sewer and water services not only reinforced residential segregation but also undermined the quality of housing for Blacks in the state's leading industrial city. In 1909, a city ordinance mandated improvements in the city's sanitation services but specified that such improvements would cover the area "South and west of the blocks dense with black families."[65]

Atlanta not only neglected the sanitation needs of African American, poor, and working-class residents, but the city permitted the dumping of garbage in and around their neighborhoods. Disproportionately larger numbers of African Americans occupied the city's three districts—the first, second, and fourth—with the highest incidence of unsanitary and unsafe housing prone to disastrous flooding.[66] Despite Durham's renown as a city of homes and prosperity among urban Blacks, as historian Leslie Brown documents, late nineteenth- and early twentieth-century Durham was also an unsanitary, disease-ridden place, where undiagnosed "Durham fever" took a heavy toll on the health and well-being of the city's Black population.[67] In New Orleans, similarly unsanitary and hazardous living environments drove the city's Black death rate up from 37 per 1,000 population to 42 per 1,000 population between 1890 and 1900. At the same time, the city's white death rate declined, although only slightly from 25 to 24 per 1,000 population. In Washington, DC, Black migrants from the South swelled the city's many poor alley dwellings, numbering about 231 in 1880.

From the outset of the emancipation era, the Washington *Intelligencer* described the capital city's alley housing as generally constructed of the "cheapest lumber, covered with felt and tar." Nearly a decade later, health officials reported alley housing as "miserable dilapidated shanties, patched and filthy." Such housing, the report continued, were "unfit for human habitation." Over the next several decades, conditions for alley dwellers steadily declined compared to their street side counterparts. By 1910, the alley death rate stood at about 30 per 1,000 population to 18 per 1,000 for street residents. The infant mortality rate was even more lopsided at 373 per 1,000 for alley dwellers and 159 per 1,000 for street people.[68] Although Black urbanites were more widely dispersed across the landscape in cities in the South than in the North, they nonetheless clustered near cemeteries, industrial sites, railroads, and flood plains across the country. Almost everywhere, African Americans were also the chief "shanty" and alley dwellers. By the early twentieth century, municipal boards of health repeatedly described alley dwellings as "shanties . . . [with] leaky roofs, broken and filthy ceilings, dilapidated floors . . . [and] unfit for human habitation."[69]

Between the Civil War and World War I, an estimated 400,000 Blacks left the South. The percentage of Blacks living in the North and West increased from 7.8 percent in 1860 to about 11 percent in 1910. A few East Coast and Midwest cities, like Philadelphia, Chicago, Pittsburgh, and New York, absorbed the bulk of these newcomers, who came mainly from the Upper South and border states of Tennessee, Kentucky, Missouri, and Virginia. By 1910, New York's Black population rose to 91,700, the largest urban concentration of Blacks in the country. Philadelphia's Black population reached 84,500, the fifth largest concentration of Blacks in the country, behind the District of Columbia, New Orleans, New York, and Baltimore.[70] In the urban Northeast,

Black migrants from the South took jobs in a variety of manufacturing and nonmanufacturing sectors of the economy of New York, Philadelphia, and Boston, but migrants to the Midwest moved almost exclusively into the mass production industries. They took the hottest, heaviest, and lowest-paying jobs at the cellar of the industrial workforce; labored primarily as general laborers rather than factory operatives; and took housing in the most dilapidated, unhealthy, and crowded sections of the urban housing market.

The initial wave of newcomers moved into neighborhoods within or adjacent to the cities' designated "red light" or "vice" districts. Replete with an underground economy of gambling, brothels, dance halls, and bootlegging establishments, these areas often received such local designations as the "bad lands." By the beginning of World War I, however, Progressive Era reformers had organized movements to demolish the so-called vice districts and drove them deeper into expanding African American communities within the city.[71] According to the Atlanta University "Conference for the Study of the Negro Problems," African Americans lived in areas where TB or "consumption" had emerged as the "greatest enemy of the black race." At the turn of the twentieth century, the TB rate of African Americans nearly tripled the rate of whites. TB was an especially troubling disease for African Americans because it tended to strike down victims in the middle-age prime, the "most productive phase of their life." David McBride explains that TB is an infectious disease that is "usually spread by inhalation of airborne droplets secreted by persons usually severely diseased who have [the germ] tubercle bacilli in their sputum. Causal pathogens for TB had been identified by the historic bacteria laboratory research of [Dr. Robert] Koch and his generation" of medical investigators. Between 1884 and 1900, TB deaths for African Americans in Boston, Washington, DC, Baltimore, and New York City ranged from a low of 448 to a high of 742 per 100,000 population compared to an average of 174 for whites in the same cities. Southern cities reported somewhat lower African American deaths, on average, from TB than cities in the North, but Blacks nonetheless had considerably higher death rates from the disease than their white counterparts in the South.[72]

In addition to TB and other diseases associated with their earlier lives as bondmen and women, emancipation-era African Americans confronted the ravages of two newly recognized though not entirely new dietary-related illnesses—pellagra and rickets—brought on, respectively, by deficiencies of niacin and calcium in the diet. Until the early twentieth century, pellagra was considered a Black infectious disease. Symptoms include "deep skin eruptions" followed by diarrhea, dementia, and death for large numbers of victims (some estimated 40 percent). However, after about 1906, when the corn-processing industry started to remove niacin from the product, white cases of pellagra multiplied, and the disease gained widespread recognition as a product of a dietary deficiency rather than a contagious disease. Even more so than in rural areas (where Blacks had greater access to garden crops), Black urbanites consumed diets deficient in fresh meats, milk, eggs, fruits, and vegetables.[73]

Large numbers of African Americans also suffered from sickle cell anemia, characterized by excessive pain, bruising of the skin, anemia, and "extensive sores." Unlike most other diseases among Black people, sickle cell anemia resulted from a genetic disorder identified by "many pear-shaped and elongated forms" in the blood. While some whites developed the sickle cell anemia, popular and even medical professionals insisted on treating this disease as a Black affliction and reinforced the notion of the inherent "inferiority" of Black people.[74]

As rural, semirural, and urban industrial labor and living conditions took their toll on the lives of Black workers and their families, the mainstream white medical establishment continued to view African Americans as genetically prone toward physical weakness, susceptibility to disease, and slated for eventual extinction as a people. The white medical profession continued to emphasize making Black bodies fit for work, labor, and profits in a racialized capitalist political economy. But postbellum African Americans did not quietly accept the spread of disease and racist medical science and healing practices. They resisted the intellectual underpinnings as well as the racial practices of the American medical profession. Challenges to medical segregation and discrimination were deeply rooted in the history of grassroots African American resistance to inequality of diagnoses and treatment of disease extending back to the antebellum years and earlier. Most important, however, African Americans' health and health care struggles revealed their firm determination to rebuild and even expand their earlier pre–Civil War health care system.

Rebuilding and Expanding the Black Health System

Emancipation-era Black people used a variety of old and new strategies for shaping the terms on which they lived, worked, and secured medical care for themselves and their families. They reestablished access to their historic garden plots for growing their own food and extended their folk healing practices, especially midwifery, into the new century. Most importantly, they expanded their roster of college- and university-trained medical profession-als. By the onset of World War I, they had organized a variety of nurse train-ing schools, small hospitals, and "local health and social hygiene campaigns." But they did not act entirely alone. This remarkable achievement was partly a product of interracial cooperation among Black and white health care pro-fessionals and philanthropists.[75]

Reconstruction of the Black health care system was by no means a fully harmonious interracial and intraracial organizing process. College- and university-trained medical professionals took the lead in rebuilding the Af-rican American medical infrastructure. For their part, however, poor and working-class Black men and women root doctors, conjurers, and midwives faced increasing pressure within and outside the Black community to termi-nate their services. They fought an uphill but ultimately losing battle against both the white supremacist medical system and the growing professional-ization of the Black medical system. Even so, partly because of the continu-ing dearth of Black physicians and the high cost of physician care, midwives continued to deliver most babies in poor and working-class Black rural and urban communities well into the twentieth century.[76]

The postbellum reconstruction of Black health care entailed an ongoing and dynamic interaction between medical apartheid, the expanding Black medical profession, and the persistence of the grassroots informal Black folk medical tradition. Historian Gretchen Long creatively documents these com-plicated cross-currents in the medical struggles of three African American healers from the outset of the emancipation era through the late nineteenth century. The careers of John Donaldson of Austin, Texas; Moses Camplin of Charleston, South Carolina; and Alexander Augustus of Washington, DC, illuminate three paths forward in the post–Civil War rebuilding of the Black medical system.[77]

Alternative Paths toward Rebuilding the Black Health System

In 1866, John Donaldson, an ex-slave and Black folk medical practitioner, wrote a letter to General Oliver Howard, head of the federal Freedmen's Bureau. Because he was not a legally certified physician, Donaldson com-plained that the white bureau agent had encouraged Black residents not to pay him for medical services that he had provided on a "for fee" basis. In his own words, Donaldson explained that the agent "said to freedmen for despite he's got no license; Nor no Deplomer. Don't pay him."[78] Donaldson asked the bureau chief to intervene on his behalf and help him collect money from patients whom he had treated according to their prior agreement or contract.

A traditional healer who continued to practice his craft in the first years after freedom, Donaldson acknowledged that he had "no license; Nor no Deplomer," but he insisted that he was a legitimate physician who honorably served his people, a practice that he had pursued before the Civil War. Indeed, according to his letter, the Freedmen's Bureau had hired a white doctor to address the health needs of the newly emancipated Black population and forced him out of business by refusing to help him collect money from his patients. Donaldson vigorously defended his medical knowledge as a doctor against the established standard of the modern Euro-American medical establishment: "I am not a Mineral physician, Professionally. I can use it but it is not good in this climate [central Texas]. I use rather herb. My father had ME Learned under an Indian phys. If any Man say that I ever lost a case, he is vast mistaken."[79] By 1880, the US Census listed Donaldson as a "laborer," but he amended the census document by writing "Dr." for "doctor" above his name on the form. Donaldson's career clearly revealed the traditional Black healer under siege after freedom.

An emerging "better class" of African Americans supported the Freedmen's Bureau and its assault on Donaldson's medical practice. Their responses highlight the growing pressure on folk healers from an emerging Black middle class. In the summer of 1866, the freedmen's organization, the Texas Lawyer Lege of Liberty, wrote to the national office of the Freemen's Bureau. The letter declared that we "were glad to find that we have friends in Washington. . . . Mr. John Donaldson . . . is a pest. . . . He passes as a quack Doctor and we are sure his complaint is for his self."[80] Yet, even the bureau agents who testified against Donaldson's medical practice conceded that he received substantial support among poor and working-class Black patients. Some of these patients had no doubt consulted Donaldson before and during the war and now continued to patronize his medical service. While the bureau ordinarily insisted that newly emancipated people honor their contracts with former slave owners, it overtly worked to deprive a folk physician of his livelihood by encouraging freed people to violate their agreement with him. The bureau also belittled his medical knowledge. One bureau agent wrote that if Donaldson was so "able to conjure diseases out of his patients bodies, he ought to be able also to conjure his fees out of their pockets, without the interference of the Bureau."[81]

Moses Camplin, another ex-slave physician, had been trained by a prominent white surgeon in Charleston, South Carolina. Two weeks after gaining his freedom in 1865, Camplin set up his own independent medical practice among the city's Black population. During the summer of 1866, Camplin wrote a letter to the Freedmen's Bureau seeking help to reopen his practice after hostile municipal and medical officials closed his office. Camplin explained that he had received training and worked in the medical office of Dr. Thomas L. Ogier, a prominent and well-connected Charleston physician. As an enslaved man, he described how he had practiced medicine among his people without hindrance. He asked the bureau to overturn the city's decision to close his office on the premise that he lacked formal medical school training. Camplin firmly advanced his case that racial "prejudice" and not inadequate training had barred him from the medical field. In his own words, he said, "only my Color and prejudice against me, and not my ability," were responsible for closing his practice.

Furthermore, Camplin cited examples of well-known white physicians allowed to practice without formal medical school training. "Dr. Smythe and others," he said, "practice medicine here, over 20 years, who never been in any medical college and who never received a Diploma from any medical Board in the world—and because they were white they was allowed to practice medicine and to give certification in death without *molestation* from any authority, State, or City."[82] In addition, Camplin reported how he sought to enroll in the South Carolina Medical College to satisfy the demands made on him, but the dean of the college informed him in no uncertain terms that "the Medical College will not admit colored men to its benefit, nor will the medical Board License any colored person to practice medicine in the State of So. Ca."[83]

Unlike the case of Donaldson, the federal Freedmen's Bureau sided with Camplin and ordered the reinstatement of his medical practice. The city rejected the bureau's decision and continued to obstruct Camplin's medical practice. However, with bureau and widespread community support, Camplin was able to reopen his practice despite the city's effort to close him down. Camplin's experience nonetheless underscored the difficult path that well-educated Black medical professionals would have to travel before they could practice medicine during the early postbellum and Jim Crow era. The case of Alexander Augustus provides yet another case study of the numerous obstacles that confronted African Americans in their efforts to rebuild their health care system during the first generation of freedom, whether formerly enslaved or free Blacks.

During the Civil War years, Alexander Augustus, another African American doctor, wrote to the Freedmen's Bureau asking for assistance to remove racial barriers that limited his ability to practice medicine. In contrast to both Camplin and Donaldson, Augustus secured his freedom before the Civil War. He had also earned his medical degree from Trinity College in Toronto, Canada, in 1856. But his status as a free African American did not shield him from the destructive impact of the color line in the American health care system. His formal training in the medical field allowed him to obtain a job as surgeon in the Union Army. In 1863, when Augustus received appointment as head surgeon of the US Colored Troops, the white doctors rebelled against his supervision. In an angry letter to Freedmen's Bureau and military officials, the white employees under his authority vehemently protested: "We cannot in any cause, willingly compromise what we consider a proper self-respect . . . service, as subordinate to a colored officer. We therefore most respectfully, yet earnestly, request that this . . . most unpleasant relationship . . . be terminated."[84]

The Medical Division promptly removed Augustus from his surgical position to a new job in Baltimore. In his new post, he carried out routine physicals on new Black recruits in the Union Army. Adding insult to injury, he was compensated at the same pay as his recruits. Only his petition to the US Senate resulted in an adjustment to his pay. Following the Civil War, Augustus received an appointment at Camp Barker and later became a doctor and faculty member when Freedmen's Hospital became the medical school for Howard University. Although trained in the mainstream conventions of modern medicine, Alexander Augustus's medical career revealed yet another permutation on the many racialized obstacles that would beset the African American community as it moved to rebuild its shattered health care system following the Civil War.

Against the broader backdrop of numerous class and racial barriers on their access to equal medical school training and treatment of disease, African Americans worked hard to reestablish and expand their prewar system for healing themselves. As suggested by the diverse experiences of Augustus, Camplin, and Donaldson, efforts to reconstruct the Black medical system had roots in the war years. Even as the war picked up steam and the government gradually appropriated resources for the wartime health needs of Black people, African Americans did not wait for government and wartime aid before they set about trying to cure themselves. They soon transformed some of the "contraband" camps into virtual wartime African American communities. These otherwise makeshift settlements provided the spatial context for the development of "networks of self-help." These networks allowed displaced Black families and communities to acquire necessary food, clothing, shelter, and a degree of access to folk as well as mainstream medical practices. They also helped African Americans build bridges to the social services of established Black and white voluntary organizations like the American Missionary Association that sent volunteers into the war zone.[85]

Reestablishing Old and Initiating New Institutional Health Movements

In the postbellum and Jim Crow eras, African Americans intensified efforts to reestablish their own viable health care system in the aftermath of war. As freed men and women reestablished themselves on the land, vegetable gardens played a major role in postbellum efforts to supplement their diets and counter certain vitamin deficiencies associated with the so-called three Ms: "meal, meat, and molasses." Closely aligned with the Civil War's disruption of the antebellum Black health care system, the rebellion initially also disconnected many Blacks from this historic resource. But it soon resurfaced and expanded within the context of the sharecropping system in which Black families took a greater hand in managing their own labor within the limits of sharecrop and tenant contracts. Even the poorest sharecroppers and tenant farmers maintained some crops for their own subsistence, but the fruits of these plots varied significantly from place to place, especially among the small number of Black landowners and the tenant farmers. In her innovative study of Promised Land, historian Elizabeth Rauh Bethel compared the garden produce of one tenant family (the Lites) with that of a small landowning family (Letmans) and concluded that the Letman table was "high in protein and relatively well balanced," including fresh fruits and vegetables, while the Lites "existed on cornbread, greens, fatback, and molasses, food high in calories but low in nutritional value and not able to [fully] support the physical demands of labor-intensive farming."[86]

As African Americans struggled to reestablish access to life-giving vegetable gardens and farm produce for their own consumption and health, they also intensified the health service activities of their religious, social welfare, fraternal, and mutual benefit organizations and clubs.[87] Black public health, civic leaders, and grassroots activists knitted together what medical historian David McBride describes as a massive network of "public health voluntarism." This extensive self-help medical structure included "public-oriented" professional associations, medical schools, and nurse training programs and facilities.[88] In her study, *Sick and Tired of Being Sick and Tired*, historian Susan L. Smith persuasively argued that Black women's health work "laid the community roots of public health work." According to Smith, this work emerged midway between the work of "personal charity and professional social work" and shaped the "direction of social welfare during the Progressive Era." In her view, Black women played a pivotal role in the South's adoption of public health services as a public policy.[89]

Women's clubs and self-help groups like the Phillis Wheatley Club of New Orleans, the Dorchester Home in Dorchester, Massachusetts, and the Lucy Brown Club of Charleston, South Carolina, provided indispensable support to the health care organizing campaigns within African American communities. In October 1896, the Phillis Wheatly Club launched the Phillis Wheatley Sanitarium and Training School for Nurses in the Crescent City. From its inception, this institution aimed "to serve the health-care needs of black New Orleans and to provide facilities for the training of black health care personnel." All-male clubs also pitched in to advance the health care of African Americans as the Jim Crow system of segregation and exclusion intensified. In 1905, in Savannah, Georgia, the Men's Sunday Club held meetings to address community-wide health issues, among numerous other concerns. Some 200 people regularly attended these meetings. According to the club's president Monroe N. Work, the club demonstrated that the "gospel of health could be carried directly to the colored people and that they were ready to hear and put into practice" what they learned.[90]

Fraternal orders and mutual benefit societies also launched their own special health campaigns to help alleviate the suffering not only of their members but of the larger Black community. In 1908, in Hot Springs, Arkansas, the local chapter of the African American Knights of Pythia established a "bathhouse and sanitorium" where thousands of Black residents sought "water care" to treat certain ailments. Closely intertwined with the health work of the Black churches, activists also organized African American anti-TB leagues in Norfolk, Portsmouth, and Richmond, Virginia. The Richmond league enthusiastically reported on its extensive program of anti-TB activities:

The third Sunday in January, 1910 was observed as tuberculosis day.
A sermon on tuberculosis was preached in nearly every colored church in Richmond and literature bearing on the subject was distributed. . . .
A registered nurse, as chairman, did very A [quality] work by affiliating with the city health authorities in hunting up tubercular patients and providing proper treatment. The committee divided the city into districts and nurses were assigned to each. . . . Food, clothing,

medicine, and even fuel has been furnished for the sick. . . . The membership of the league is about four hundred.[91]

Varieties of self-help organizations, particularly women's clubs, fueled the rise of spirited independent Black hospital and nurse training school movements across the country during the final decade of the nineteenth century and the opening years of the twentieth century. These movements were partly inspired by the pioneering work of Freedmen's Hospital at Howard University in Washington, DC. Freedmen's Hospital, the nation's leading Black medical college, had its beginnings in the work of the Freedmen's Bureau following the Civil War, when the federal government transformed Camp Barker, a contraband camp, into a hospital for freed men and women and their families. In July 1868, however, federal financial support for the facility came to an end, but the hospital continued service when bureau head Oliver Howard transferred it to the new Howard University medical department. Rather than being a federally funded effort, however, the hospital received its principal funding from a special "hospital tax" levied on Black workers and "on the profits from freedmen's agriculture." As historian Gretchen Long makes clear, Freedmen's Hospital "was neither a charity nor even a purely government enterprise. It was funded and maintained by money earned and paid involuntarily by freedmen, and later it became crucial in training African American doctors through its connections with the Howard University medical department."[92]

Black workers by no means unanimously embraced the involuntary hospital tax as a common good. Some Black workers protested the tax as a violation of their rights as free citizens. A group of African American cooks, for example, petitioned the secretary of war to terminate the tax. In their appeal, they declared that they represented "A Portion of that Class of Colored Men (Termed free) And Pretending as We Do To have Some faint Conceptions of the value of our labor." Such protests notwithstanding, the hospital tax underscored the critical role that the earnings and labor of poor and working-class Blacks would play in rebuilding the Black medical infrastructure nationwide. While the labor and earnings of the Black working class fueled the growth of Howard's medical school, college- and university-trained Black physicians like Charles Purvis and Colonel Alexander T. Augustus (discussed previously) and their white allies like Robert Reyburn and others provided early institutional leadership for the school. By the late 1870s, Freedmen's Hospital served about 2,270 outpatients and wrote an estimated 4,000 prescriptions for drug treatments.[93]

As the nation's earliest Black hospital, Freedmen's Hospital at Howard University emerged as a great "beacon" for the spread of the Black hospital movement. Meharry Medical College, founded in Nashville, Tennessee, in 1876, emerged as the second most prominent Black medical school in the country. While Howard attracted a multinational student body, Meharry was the first Black medical school devoted solely to the training of African American physicians. By 1906, Black health activists had established forty voluntary hospitals, five medical schools, and a plethora of "smaller health centers." Six years later, the number of health care centers had increased to sixty-five, mostly in Southern towns and cities. In rural areas of the South, public and private medical facilities provided little or no help for African Americans. If rural Blacks required hospitalization, they had to travel to a hospital in nearby towns or cities with a "Jim Crow ward." Many of them were not so eager to seek help from white hospitals. Remembering the regular use of Black bodies for medical experimentation before emancipation, they were reluctant to put themselves at risk of such experimentation in the era of freedom.[94]

Leading Black-controlled hospitals and nursing schools included most notably Provident Hospital and Nurse Training School in Chicago; Tuskegee Institute and Nurse Training School in Alabama; and the Frederick Douglass Memorial Hospital and Training School in Philadelphia. Black hospitals and nurse training programs powered the expansion of Black physicians nationwide from under 1,000 in 1890 to over 3,400 in 1910. The number of Black nurses also expanded, but nurses faced an even steeper climb than Black men into the ranks of professional medical service during the period.[95] In August 1879, Mary E. Mahoney became the first Black nurse to graduate from a certified all-white nursing school. She received her degree from the New England Hospital for Women and Children in Boston. The school's charter specified that only one Black and one Jewish student would be accepted into the school each year.

By the turn of the twentieth century, only five other Black women had gained their degrees from the institution. But most other nurse training programs in the country excluded Black women. The Black hospital and nurse training movement was, however, instrumental in increasing the number of Black nurses to over 2,400 in 1910. Indeed, the movement not only hoped to expand the ranks of Black nurses and provide opportunities for Black physicians to serve their patients but also to inculcate certain values into the young graduates of these programs—particularly a profound resolve to address the health and well-being of the African American community. Eminent historian Darlene Clark Hine underscored this agenda in her pioneering study,

Black Women in White: "What these hospital training schools seemed to have imparted most effectively to their graduates was a sense of commitment to and responsibility for the black community and its health-care institutions. The nurses trained in these schools were expected to owe primary allegiance to black people."[96]

Backed up by broad cross-sections of Black urban communities, African American hospitals and nurse training programs emerged under the dynamic leadership of predominantly male university-trained Black physicians. Born in Hollidaysburg, Pennsylvania, the Black surgeon Dr. Daniel Hale Williams spearheaded the formation of Provident Hospital and Nurse Training School in Chicago in 1891. The son of a barber and "well-to-do landowner" and a mother who apparently maintained the home without the necessity of entering the paid labor force, Williams received his MD degree from the Chicago Medical College and postdoctoral training at Mercy Hospital, a Catholic institution in the city. He soon set up a well-respected and lucrative interracial medical practice and would gain renown for performing one of the first successful open heart operations.

Although Williams led the founding of Provident Hospital, the club woman and journalist Fannie Barrier Williams (no relation to the surgeon and founder) organized the fundraising drive for the facility. Under her leadership, the financial campaign raised over $2,000 from Black and white donors. Mrs. Cara Scott Pond, also a club woman, raised another $1,300 for the effort. Other community members, mostly women, donated gifts in kind, including "a parlor stove, a clothes wringer, chiffon lace for nurse's caps, books, and portraits." In 1912, largely as a result of the energetic fundraising activities of Black women, Provident reported "no debts, an endowment of $50,000 [of which $45,000 had been donated by Blacks], and a plant valued at $125,000."

Dr. Williams vigorously urged African Americans to stop "wasting time trying to effect changes or modifications" in white institutions "unfriendly to us, but rather let us seek to promote the doctrine of helping and stimulating our race." At the same time, he nonetheless insisted on making Provident an interracial organization that would welcome whites as well as Blacks. As historian Vanessa Northington Gamble concludes, Provident's founder originally "perceived the hospital not as an exclusively black enterprise, but as an interracial one that would not practice racial discrimination with regard to staff privileges, nurse training school applicants, and the admission of patients."[97]

Moved by the exclusion of Black nurses from Philadelphia's white nurse training programs, Dr. Nathan Francis Mossell headed the formation of the Frederick Douglass Memorial Hospital. Born in Hamilton, Ontario, to Black American parents who migrated to Canada from Baltimore, Mossell received his undergraduate education from Lincoln University in Pennsylvania; his MD degree from the University of Pennsylvania; and postgraduate training at London's well-regarded Guy's Hospital and the city's St. Thomas Hospital. Blocked from practicing in the city's white hospital, on June 25, 1895, he issued a call for Black physicians and leading ministers to join him in launching "a separate hospital where black doctors could enjoy staff, consulting, and admitting privileges, black patients could receive cure[s], and black women could enter nursing training." Initially, Frederick Douglass Memorial Hospital occupied a three-story house. However, in 1908, following a long and intensive fundraising campaign, the hospital opened for patients at 1512 Lombard Street. Furthermore, as Mossell put it, Frederick Douglass Memorial Hospital "would not discriminate" on the basis of race, admission, employment, training or patient treatment. The hospital included whites in planning, board membership, and financial campaigns.[98]

As suggested by the health-organizing activities of Black club women and physicians Daniel Hale Williams and Nathan Francis Mossell, the Black health care movement was by no means all-Black. It entailed substantial interracial alliances with sympathetic Euro-American philanthropic elites. White allies and supporters of Black hospital and nursing school campaigns included, most notably, John D. Rockefeller, Andrew Carnegie, Julius Rosenwald, and the Duke family of Durham, North Carolina. In 1901, under ongoing pressure from Aaron M. Moore, the only Black physician in the town, and John Merrick, the highly successful barber, entrepreneur, and founder of North Carolina Mutual insurance company, the Duke family financed the building of Durham's Lincoln Hospital for Blacks and, somewhat later, the nursing school. Philanthropic supporters of African American health care campaigns included significant numbers of activist white women as well as men. As early as 1881, John D. Rockefeller and his wife Laura Spelman financed the founding of the Atlanta Baptist Female Seminary, later renamed Spelman College. But the nursing school itself was not established until 1886. It became "the first two-year program leading to a diploma in nursing established within an academic institution." In 1901, the Atlanta campus also opened a thirty-one-bed hospital "to serve as a school infirmary and practice facility for the student nurses."[99]

Somewhat similar to Laura Spelman, New Englander Alice Mabel Bacon founded the Dixie Hospital Training School for nurses in Hampton, Virginia, in 1891. While some male advocates of nurses training accented the role that this training could play in making the young women "better wives" and helpers for Black doctors, Bacon emphasized nurse training as neither a route to better wifery or service to Black physicians per se, but rather as a route to "the delivery of better health care for black people and the simultaneous production of autonomous professionals." Five white women also led the founding of St. Agnes Hospital and nurse training school in Raleigh, North Carolina. They established the school in a private residence on the campus of the city's St. Augustine College for Negroes.[100]

African American hospitals and nurse training schools varied significantly from place to place, depending on the local political economy and network of alliances that African Americans were able to forge with their white supporters as well as the dynamics of class, social, and political relations within the nearby African American communities. The contrast between the two earliest Black medical schools, Howard and Meharry, captures some of the key differences between African American hospitals and medical education programs during the heyday of Jim Crow. The two schools were different but complementary institutions. Howard firmly embraced the standards of the nation's leading white medical schools, while Meharry embraced a more grassroots "organic" relationship to the local Black community. Under the leadership of its white faculty and with its "multinational and multicultural" student body, Howard "was very aware of and sensitive to medical education's new scientific trends and movements toward specialization." Conversely, Meharry, with its focus on training Black medical professionals, would "eventually train and graduate more Black physicians than any other institution in the world." According to medical historians Byrd and Clayton, Meharry accomplished this feat by "producing grassroots, primary care-oriented practitioners with folksy manners and the common touch, almost deceptively combining professional skills and new medical technology with the imagery of the Old South's Black healer roots."[101]

Despite important differences among Black medical schools, Black medical professionals, educators, and activists gradually came together to build a greater sense of cohesiveness, common goals, and community across institutions. This work gained highly organized expression with the creation of the National Medical Association (NMA) in 1895, the National Association of Colored Graduate Nurses in 1908, and the *Journal of the National Medical Association* in 1909. Black physicians established the NMA to combat racial discrimination in the American Medical Association. Local chapters of the organization spread across the country as the number of Black physicians gradually increased. The NMA did not emerge from thin air. It built upon a network of local medical associations that had emerged during the 1880s and early 1890s. Earlier Black medical associations included the Tennessee Colored Medical Association (1880); the Medico-Chirurgical Society of the District of Columbia (1884); the Old North State Medical Society of North Carolina; and the Association of Physicians, Dentists, and Pharmacists of Georgia (1893). By 1892, African American physicians had also launched the nation's first Black medical journal, the *Medical and Surgical Observer*. This pioneering medical organ also announced the call for a meeting to form a national Black medical association.[102]

The founding of the NMA at the First Congregational Church in Atlanta in 1895 coincided with the city's famous international cotton exposition, the death of renown abolitionist Frederick Douglass, and the rise of Booker T. Washington to prominence following his famous Atlanta Compromise Address. The NMA not only aimed to organize Black medical professionals. It also insisted on working to "insure progressiveness in the profession" and, perhaps most important, to "improve living conditions among the Negro people by teaching them the *simple rules of health*." Membership in the NMA rose from under 50 or so at its founding to over 500 by 1912. The NMA also used its professional publication, the *Journal of the National Medical Association* (*JNMA*), to serve "the interests of Negro physicians, surgeons, dentists and pharmacists" and to "raise the public's consciousness of preventive health measures."

As Dr. John A. Kenney, Tuskegee Institute's medical director, put it, the *JNMA* "is also planned and written that it is of general interest to nurses, teachers, ministers, and any intelligent laymen who are interested in the progress of the race." These organizations emerged during the consolidation of the Jim Crow order, but they were not solely a response to the racially exclusionary ideas and practices of the segregationist system. Medical historian Vanessa Northington Gamble forcefully argues that the Black hospital movement was also a product of the African American community's "longstanding tradition of providing for its members."[103]

African Americans not only set about forging a public health movement to cure themselves, they also gave substantial attention to developing alternative nonracial interpretations of infectious diseases. Among these Black physicians who challenged the racial paradigm were Dr. Daniel Hale Williams; Dr. Charles V. Roman, a president of the NMA; and the authors of essays appearing in publications of the Atlanta University Conference, among other outlets for writing on medicine and health issues. In 1900, Williams published an essay challenging the "almost universal" notion among white surgeons "that colored women did not have ovarian tumors." Similarly, as a professor of medicine at Meharry Medical College, Roman published a book titled *American Civilization and the Negro—The Afro-American in Relation to National Progress* (1916). Roman declared that "if he [the Negro] is susceptible to disease (as tuberculosis), he is a weakling; if he is not susceptible (as hookworm), he is a menace."

At the 1906 Atlanta University Conference on the Study of Negro Problems, attendees heard papers delivered by a rising cohort of interracial antiracist scholars and educators, including Monroe N. Work, Franz Boas, and Herbert Miller. As historian David McBride noted, these presenters "contested the evolutionist idea of an amorphous, inferior Negro race." For his part, Dr. Kenney of the Tuskegee Institute underscored the determination of African Americans to launch their own self-help movement in the face of white skepticism about their capacity to improve their health status and avoid extinction. "Without quibbling over such academic questions as whether the Negro is dying as rapidly as some other people . . . the race is realizing that its death-rate is high; that certain diseases are taking more than their toll of human life from its ranks, and that many of these diseases are preventable. With this realization, many Negroes have set to work to improve their living conditions and reduce mortality."[104]

As African Americans escalated their movements toward building their own medical schools, journals, and nurse training programs, the US medical profession intensified its push to professionalize and control standards for the practice of medicine. At the opening of the new century, the field had already eliminated the so-called quacks ("homeopaths, hydrotherapists, and the like") from their ranks. It now turned toward eradicating what it deemed "poorly trained and incompetent" physicians, whatever degrees or educational credentials such practitioners presented as proof of their professionalism. Organized physicians—namely, the American Medical Association (AMA)—secured financial and moral support for this undertaking from leading philanthropic organizations, foundations, and medical schools as well as from the American Association of Medical Colleges, the AMA's own Council on Medical Education, and most importantly, the Carnegie Foundation.[105]

Changing standards for the practice of medicine undercut the African American medical infrastructure and reinforced the debilitating impact of neglect. In 1904, the AMA established a new Council on Medical Education and set about reforming the medical profession as practiced in the United States. It called for a rigorous regimen of training to become a state-certified physician, a process that doctors controlled through the AMA. The new standard called for a minimum of four years of high school, four years of formal medical training, another year of hospital internship, and passage of a state licensing exam to practice medicine. Published in 1910, the Flexner Report, funded by the Carnegie Foundation, established the new standard for medical education in the United States and Canada. The report took the name of its principal researcher, Abraham Flexner—a professional educator with higher education degrees (but not the PhD) from Johns Hopkins, Harvard, and the University of Berlin. The Flexner Report, combined with the rising costs of health care, led to the closure of numerous hospitals and drove down the number of practicing physicians. African American medical professionals and their Black clients were hardest hit.[106]

The Flexner Report had a profound effect on the medical education of African Americans. It severely curtailed the expansion of the segregated Black medical infrastructure without opening the door to equal access to the nation's all-white medical establishment. Among the seven African American schools surveyed by Flexner, only two (Howard and Meharry) received a passing grade; one received a marginal pass, and the remainder received a failing grade. Flexner visited scores of medical schools across the country, but he seemed especially abrasive in upbraiding Black schools for failing to meet the emerging standards that the AMA had set for medical education. In one case, he roundly criticized the Knoxville Medical College for housing its college "above a funeral parlor" and concluded that the institution's promotional materials provided "misrepresentations from cover to cover."[107]

In a section of the report titled "The Medical Education of the Negro," Flexner reinforced the prevailing racist wisdom regarding Black education during the era of white supremacist medical thought and practices. He supported the notion of a distinct medical education for aspiring young Blacks seeking to enter the medical field as physicians and nurses, but he called for a clear color divide. Flexner suggested that African American medical schools provide opportunities for "the more promising of their race . . . to receive a substantial education in which *hygiene rather than surgery, for example, is strongly accentuated.*"[108]

By recommending the exclusion of African Americans from the dynamic, lucrative, and prestigious surgical field, the Flexner Report buoyed the system of medical apartheid and set the stage for the severe curtailment of Black medical schools, nurse training programs, and quality health care services for Black people during the era of the Great Migration. Before the Flexner Report, African Americans had reported seven medical schools serving Black doctors and nurses. Following World War I, that number dropped to only two medical schools serving the African American community—Howard University in the District of Columbia and Meharry Medical College in Nashville, Tennessee. Meanwhile, the Carnegie and Rockefeller Foundations provided increasing support to leading white medical schools that enthusiastically adopted the recommendations and requirements of the Flexner Report.[109]

Conclusion

The advent of the Civil War and the emancipation of some 4 million enslaved people dramatically changed the socioeconomic, political, and institutional foundation of African American health and health care. For the first time in the nation's history, people of African descent could lay legal claim to full citizenship rights, but the postbellum rise of the white supremacist order and its unjust labor system exposed Black people to the sharpest edges of disease and recurring epidemics during the emancipation era. Building upon the legacy of their early nineteenth-century forebears, postbellum African Americans forged a variety of responses to the health, housing, and labor challenges of the new system of medical apartheid.

Their strategies for improving their health included the ongoing cultivation of vegetable gardens; the expansion of community-based medical services under the auspices of women's clubs and religious, fraternal, and mutual benefit societies; and the development of vibrant independent Black hospital and nurse training movements. These efforts established the institutional framework for the rise of the Modern Medical Black Freedom Struggle during the industrial age. By the beginning of World War I, however, growing numbers of Black workers and their families from the South embraced the Great Migration to urban industrial America as another potent weapon in their fight against medical inequality and in pursuit of better health and well-being for their communities. These issues are explored in chapter 3.

CHAPTER THREE

Industrial Era

The Great Migration and the transformation of Black people into a predominantly urban population opened up new possibilities for better jobs, health, and living conditions during the industrial age. But racial disparities in the incidence of disease, suffering, and death persisted and even intensified. These disparities were deeply rooted in the movement of African Americans into the most dangerous and unhealthy jobs, housing, and living conditions in the industrial city. Equally and perhaps most important, they were also a product of racial discrimination, neglect, and the exclusion of African Americans from much-needed medical care in the nation's segregated and unequal Jim Crow era medical establishment. During the era of the Great Migration, the prewar expansion of the African American medical infrastructure came under increasing assault, partly from a dramatic shift in state-mandated requirements for the practice of medicine as driven by the American Medical Association (AMA). Assaults on the Black health care system had their origins in changes that had transpired on the eve of World War I, but they would play out in their most destructive form in the wake of the Great Migration during the years between the world wars and their aftermath.

Building upon what historical sociologist Alondra Nelson describes as "the long medical civil rights movement," this chapter examines how industrial-era Black communities not only continued to provide for their own health care needs but also waged a concerted battle against medical apartheid. By the late twentieth century, their efforts resulted in the fall of the segregated medical order along with the collapse of the Jim Crow political economy, politics, and institutions. These changes represented a major victory for dynamic cross-class and interracial movements within the African American community, but internal tensions along class lines did not disappear.

Many poor and working-class Blacks retained their ties to earlier folk medicine beliefs and practices. Black medical professionals and their white allies repeatedly decried such beliefs as hindrances to the delivery of modern medicine to the most vulnerable segments of the Black urban community. Industrial-era Black medical history not only took place against the backdrop of persistent forms of class and racial inequality in African American life. It also unfolded during a moment of extraordinary hope and promise for a new life of health and well-being for African Americans, their families, and their communities as the Great Migration ran its course. This chapter continues to expose the ways racist ideologies, repeatedly contested by Black agitation, gradually gave way to subtle but measurable improvements in Black health and well-being.

Moment of Hope

Beginning gradually during the late nineteenth and early twentieth century, the Great Migration escalated and ran its course in the years after World War II. By the early 1970s, an estimated 8 million Black people from the South had moved to the urban North and West. For the first time in the nation's history, large numbers of African Americans moved into the heart of the nation's urban industrial economy. They took jobs that paid Black men as much as $3.00 to $5.00 per eight-hour day compared to no more than $1.00 per day in Southern agriculture.[1]

Forging a National Migration Network

In a letter to her friend in Macon, Georgia, a recent migrant to Chicago enthusiastically wrote, "I work in Swifts packing co., in the sausage department. . . . We get $1.50 a day. . . . Tell your husband work is plentiful here and he wont have to loaf if he want to work." Another migrant to the Windy City wrote to a friend in Alabama: "Now it is true that the (col.) men are making good. Never pay less than $3.00 per day for (10) hours . . . I wish many times that you could see our people up here as they are entirely in a different light."[2] In a letter to the Urban League of Pittsburgh, one prospective migrant to the city wrote for himself and seven other Black men: "We Southern Negroes want to come to the north . . . they ain't paying a man nothing for what he do. . . . they is trying to keep us down." Even after adjustments for higher costs of living in the industrial cities, Black workers increased their earnings over Southern sharecropping and farm labor by as much as 50 to 130 percent. They often celebrated their movement into industrial jobs as a "Flight from Egypt," the "New Jerusalem," and the "Promised Land." When one group of migrants crossed the Ohio River heading north, they knelt down, prayed, and sang the hymn, "I done Come out of the Land of Egypt with the Good News."[3]

The Great Migration was not a simple South to North phenomenon. It also entailed significant movement to the urban South and West. As historian Earl

Lewis noted in his study of Black migration to Norfolk, Virginia, "more blacks migrated to southern cities between 1900 and 1920 than to Northern cities — and would continue to migrate to those cities through World War II." Unlike the urban North and South, however, only the explosive labor demands of World War II attracted massive Black migration from the South to Los Angeles, Seattle, and the San Francisco Bay Area. Much like earlier and continuing Black migration to the urban North, migrants enthusiastically mailed letters back home to Southern friends and family members, describing the urban West as "a land of milk and honey" under that "open sky."[4]

Not only did jobs and prospects for better living conditions fuel Black migration. Aspirations for higher education and improved access to health care also figured among decisions to move among many African Americans that cut across class lines. In his recent memoir *Keeping Heart: A Memoir of Family Struggle, Race, and Medicine*, Otis Trotter underscores how the prospect of obtaining advanced medical treatment for his congenital heart condition also encouraged his family to leave the southern West Virginia coalfields for a small industrial town in Ohio. As he put it, his widowed mother Thelma Trotter combined her faith in God with her confidence in modern medicine. "When we moved to Ohio in 1961, my mother had high hopes that we would experience a better way of life and that—with God's grace—I would obtain the medical care I needed for my heart."[5] Some Black women moved from the South to the North to escape violent marriage and family relations as well as racism and violent race relations. One woman, Sara Brooks, later recalled why she moved from Alabama to Cleveland, Ohio. "When he hit me," she said, "I jumped outa the bed, and when I jumped outa the bed, I just ran . . . I left the kids right there with him . . . I didn't go back."[6]

Gradual Improvements Nationwide

Certain encouraging national trends in US health and health care reinforced the perception of the industrial age as a moment of hope in African American history. Coterminous with the onset of the Great Migration, new pharmaceuticals and disease treatment protocols resulted in an overall nationwide decline in death rates for major diseases during the industrial era. Tuberculosis (TB) deaths among Blacks dropped from nearly 450 per 100,000 people in 1910 to 262 in 1920; pneumonia from nearly 260 to about 200; and heart disease from 205 to 160. In some exceptional cases, African Americans recorded lower death rates for certain diseases than their white counterparts.

In a survey of the deadly Influenza Pandemic of 1918–19 that took the lives of some 500,000 people, the US Public Health Service reported "consistently lower" death rates among African Americans than whites. Conducted by Wade Hampton Frost, a leading epidemiologist, the study investigated the spread of the disease in ten cities with populations of 25,000 to 600,000. A later study of the impact of the disease on Chicago also revealed that African Americans died at a significantly lower rate than whites during the pandemic.[7] African American life expectancy at birth also dramatically increased from only about 33 years at the outset of the new century to 46.7 years as the Great Depression got underway and to 65 years during the 1960s. The gap between Black and white life expectancy also narrowed from over 9 years in 1945 to about 7 years two decades later.[8]

In addition to improvements in their life expectancy and rates of infection for certain diseases, African Americans witnessed a gradual shift in white supremacist medical science and practice. A slowly expanding number of white physicians and public health officials embraced an anti-racist perspective that "germs know no color line." Their research repeatedly showed disproportionately high rates of disease for Blacks compared to whites, but unlike the bulk of their pre–World War I predecessors, they started to depart from beliefs about inherent racial differences as an explanation for high Black disease rates and as a rationale for limiting African American access to modern medicine, technology, and cures. As historian Samuel Kelton Roberts notes, "a new liberal racial consensus, often called interracial cooperation," gradually emerged. But their motivations for supporting an alternative perspective on race and medicine had a strong "self-interest" component. Increasing numbers among this cohort of professional healers came to believe that the status of African American health would have a profound impact on the health of white Americans, for good or for ill. And they opted to support greater medical school and nurse training programs for African Americans as a bridge between infected African American patients and modern medical science.[9]

The gradually expanding roster of anti-racist white medical professionals concurred with their African American collaborators that "germs have no color line." In 1926, a leading biologist and public health expert James A. Tobey mimicked this perspective when he said, "Microbes have not yet adopted the color line." Tobey emphasized how germs traveled a two-lane highway back and forth between Black and white communities. In articles in the *Ohio Medical Journal* and the *Child Health Bulletin*, Henry R. M. Landis, a white physician and head of social services at Philadelphia's Henry Phipps Institute, also implicitly challenged social Darwinist medical science by encouraging greater cooperation with the African American community in their fight to cure and prevent disease (including TB, syphilis, and maternal and child illnesses).[10]

Landis openly rejected the notion that African Americans were destined to die off. In his own words, he said, the "Negro is here to stay." Furthermore, he also declared that any solution to the African American health problem "other than that which recognizes that he is to continue as a permanent part of our population is preposterous." Landis then advocated assisting movements to improve the health of Black people in part, and perhaps for the most part, as a "self-interest" in our "own protection." Some formerly staunch social Darwinists, including Henry Hazen, a syphilis specialist, became firm proponents of environmentalism during the 1920s and championed programs to prevent high infant mortality rates associated with venereal disease.[11]

In 1920, African American medical professionals and their white allies gained unexpected support for their work when Louis I. Dublin, vice president and statistician for the Metropolitan Life Insurance Company, issued a research report on its African American subscribers. Dublin studied the records of some 1.7 million Black policyholders. His study confirmed that the African American death rate for various diseases were 60 percent higher than the white mortality rate. But he shocked the public health and academic world when he concluded that such racial disparities were not a product of innate Black inferiority or racial differences between Blacks and whites. He firmly argued that such inequities could be reduced by systematic programs designed to prevent and lower disease rates among African Americans.[12]

Dublin shared the results of the company's aggressive "health conservation" program—which offered free home-based nursing services and health education—with its Black and white policyholders (about 13 percent Black). According to Met-Life records for the program, between 1911, when the program got started, and 1919, African American infant mortality rate dropped by 63 percent compared to 46 percent for whites. During the same period, TB rates declined by 22 percent for Blacks and 32 percent for whites. Based upon these data, Dublin recommended greater investments in the health of Black Americans. In his words, "Colored people can profit more from such conservation work than any other race."[13]

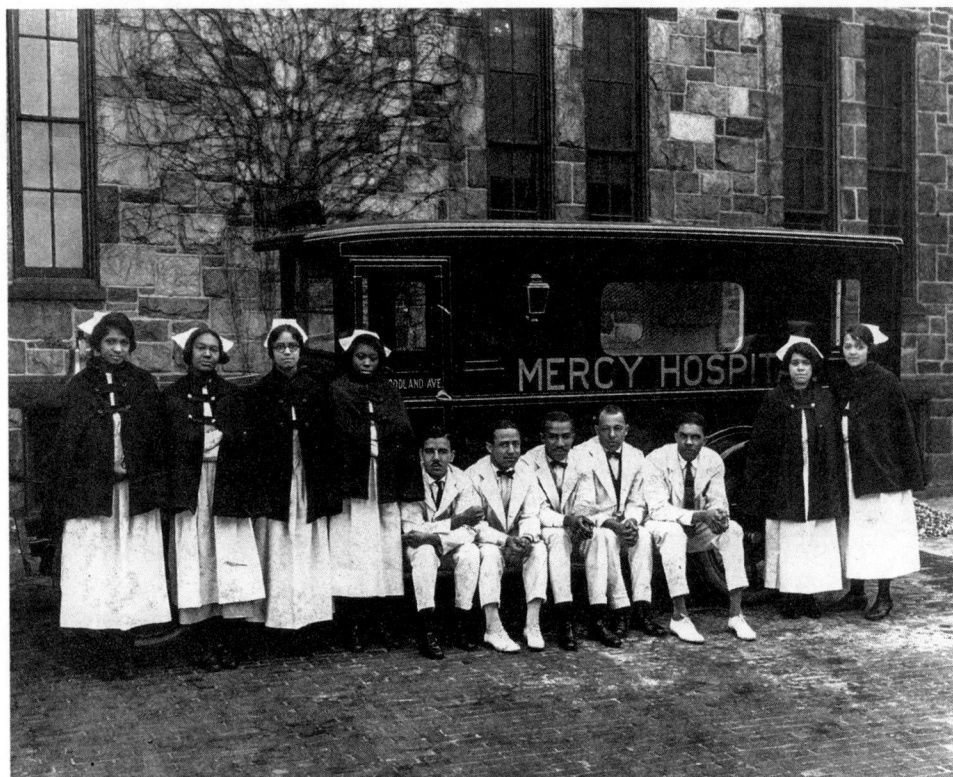

Residents and nurses, Mercy Hospital and School for Nurses, Philadelphia (1930). Courtesy of Barbara Bates Center for the Study of the History of Nursing, School of Nursing, University of Pennsylvania.

Governmental, Philanthropic, and Interracial Support for Black Health Care

Starting slowly during the 1920s, a variety of government, philanthropic, welfare, and social service organizations initiated programs designed to expand African American access to professional medical care. These activities included, most notably, modest allocations of municipal, state, federal, and philanthropic funds to support hospitals and medical centers for the treatment of Black patients and the training of Black doctors and nurses. Norfolk, Cincinnati, and Philadelphia established nationally recognized public health centers focused specifically on the medical needs of urban Black residents as the Great Migration escalated. By the stock market crash of 1929, the city of Norfolk had opened "a fully equipped public health clinic managed by Black medical and social welfare personnel." The facility not only served Blacks within the Norfolk city limits but also African Americans living in outlying small towns and rural farming communities.[14]

Similarly, in 1926, Cincinnati established the Shoemaker Health Center in the city's heavily populated African American community on the West End. The Shoemaker center became a major "multipurpose health care, medical training, and social welfare resource" for the Queen City's Black community. Based on generous funding by the Cincinnati Community Chest, the center opened the door to the citywide medical establishment to a small but significant number of Black doctors and dentists. The superintendent of the Cincinnati General Hospital and the dean of the City College of Medicine provided oversight to the African American employees of the center. For its part, in the City of Brotherly Love, the Phipps Institute medical program for Black Philadelphians had its origins in a special project aimed at encouraging tuberculosis patients to undergo "examination and treatment." Within a few years, however, the facility evolved into the institute's "Negro Health Bureau." Employing twelve Black physicians and ten Black nurses, the bureau operated four dispensaries for Black residents across the city.[15]

In 1937, following a long and intense Black hospital movement, the city of St. Louis opened Homer G. Phillips Hospital, a modern 685-bed facility for the patient care and postgraduate training for African American medical professionals. Affiliated with the Washington University School of Medicine and partly with St. Louis University, Homer G. Phillips soon gained a reputation as one of the nation's largest and most effective sites for the training of African American physicians and nurses. Since its closure in 1979, historians W. Michael Byrd and Linda Clayton doubt that its "production of excellently trained African American surgeons, orthopedic surgeons, urologists, internists, dermatologists, pediatricians, dental surgeons, nurses and allied health professions has ever been replaced." A few other cities undergoing massive Black migration—including Cleveland, Los Angeles, Memphis, and Houston—also opened public health centers for Black patients. Moreover, some of these facilities provided significant maternity and child health services under the federal Sheppard-Towner Bill.[16]

During the late 1920s and 1930s, the Julius Rosenwald Fund played a pivotal role in the development of a larger and more diverse group of Black medical professionals. Founded in 1917, the Chicago-based fund supported the building of public schools for Black children across the early twentieth-century South. During the late 1920s, however, the fund shifted its priorities to a focus on health and medical care needs of African Americans as the Great Migration to urban areas picked up steam. As medical historian David

McBride notes, Rosenwald firmly believed that the most effective "long-term solution" to the health problems confronting Black people was to increase *the number* of African American hospitals, clinics, and nursing schools for the training of Black doctors, nurses, and other health care professionals. Due to the influence of Rosenwald medical programs for African Americans, by the beginning of the Great Depression, most Southern states had employed public health nurses to serve the needs of Black people. These nurses became the "first line of defense" in medical, government, and philanthropic efforts to curtail the incidence of infectious disease within the Black community.[17]

At the same time that African Americans benefited from the increasing financial support provided by government and philanthropic sources, they also deepened their own self-help hospital movement. As the depression got underway, African Americans had established nine hospitals under the auspices of fraternal orders. The state of Arkansas claimed four of these fraternal hospitals. In 1926, they reported a membership of about 70,000 members who paid a $15 annual fee for access to medical services. By the late 1930s, in Georgia, the number of Black hospitals had increased to about thirteen, not counting four hospitals that had closed their doors.[18]

During the Great Depression, the federal government expanded support for the training of African American medical and social service professionals as part of a larger plan to prevent the spread of disease from Black to white communities. The US Public Health Service and New Deal social welfare agencies led the way. "Imperfect as they were," historian Samuel Kelton Roberts notes, "the programs erected under the New Deal had a way of inspiring faith in the power of concerted human action to remedy a variety of social problems."[19]

The New Deal federal treasury provided increasing financial support for state and local health programs, rising to some 50 percent of total expenditures during the period. African Americans embraced New Deal services as a step forward in their fight to eliminate racial barriers obstructing their path toward better health and well-being as citizens of the communities in which they lived and worked. Moreover, in the years after World War II, despite fomenting the spread of a racially segregated and unequal health system, the Hill-Burton Act increased the range of services available to Blacks over previous years. Federal law required hospitals receiving federal aid to provide funds for African American medical needs. Moreover, beginning gradually after World War II, albeit on a token basis, African

Americans slowly gained access to all-white medical school training. In 1949, the University of Arkansas admitted Edith Irby Jones to its medical school, the first African American to gain admission to an all-white medical school in the South. Other Southern medical schools slowly followed suit.[20]

As important as this progress may have been, it was insufficient to close the racial gap in the health care of Blacks and whites in urban industrial America. As African Americans registered important improvements in their health and access to medical services, they nonetheless confronted new workplace and occupational diseases as well as challenges to their emotional and psychological well-being. Decades of inequality diminished the promise of this important moment of hope in the rapidly changing but racially segregated social order. During World War I and its aftermath, managerial and labor policies concentrated Black workers in the most dangerous and unhealthy occupations. Hence, the historic making of the urban industrial Black working class entailed the arrival of new and more health issues and life-threatening diseases for the expanding and residentially segregated African American community.

Decades of Inequality

Even as African Americans celebrated the higher-paying jobs in the industrial sector compared to their experiences in Southern agriculture, they soon confronted the reality of their precarious place at the bottom tiers of the workforce. Despite its reputation as the most equitable employer of African American workers during the period, the Ford Motor Company employed Black workers almost exclusively in paint-sprayer, steel grinding, and hot and heavy foundry jobs. One Detroit automaker declared, "We hired them for this hot dirty work and we want them [to stay] there."[21] As historian Richard Walter Thomas notes, although Ford offered African Americans their greatest employment opportunities, "its foundry was a deathtrap for many black workers. The lack of safety equipment, poor ventilation, and speed-ups all contributed in one way or another to the deaths of many black workers." Autoworkers later recalled that foremen never considered "a wound as serious enough to go to first aid." After men emerged from some jobs in the foundry, one foundry worker later recalled, "They were so matted and covered with oil and dirt that no skin showed . . . the job was very rugged."[22]

In the coal mines, as discussed elsewhere, African American coal loaders continued to work in low coal seams. They had to crawl on their knees to make their way to the good coal through excessive water, bad air, and rock.[23] Meatpackers worked "where the guts and bowels all spill down. Hog kill, beef kill, beef offal, fertilizer department—those were the black jobs" in the meatpacking industry.[24] In their oral recollections of life and labor on "the killing floor," African Americans recalled dangerous and crippling conditions, made worse by insensitive foremen and supervisors. In Chicago, the Black meatpacker Philip Weightman vividly recalled one incident involving a band saw used to saw "the butts off from the picnic hams." As he remembered, "There was a band saw . . . and you know how fast they run. And when that saw happens to break, it scoots off. Vroom! If it hits anybody, it would cut 'em half in two. It had no safety on that thing northing." Weightman and two of his coworkers approached the foreman about adding a safety device on the saw, but the foreman replied, "If you don't want to work on it, you don't work; we'll find somebody else and put 'em there. It's up to you." "Oh God!" Weightman exclaimed. "So I swallowed hard on that. For a year didn't do nothing about it. Finally a guy gets his fingers sewn off."[25]

In another instance, Weightman describes "a belly bench," an area where men trimmed bacon "in a perfect trim, according to standard regulations, for it to cure and then smoke." That job entailed hard and difficult work. On this particular occasion, the company ordered a speed up of the process with a shorthanded crew that placed the available workers at risk of serious injury. Again, Weightman and a few of his comrades complained to management. "Give us some more help," they said, "because if you don't somebody's going to get cut, cut seriously." The foreman replied as anticipated, "You've been doing it all the time, you're going to continue." On a regular day-to-day basis, meatpacking firms tested the ability of the men to kill and butcher more hogs in shorter and shorter time periods. For their part, the meatpacking workers regularly complained, "They're killing [too] many hogs today, let's walk."[26]

Steelworkers manned the blast furnaces and performed the most difficult jobs while making rails for the railroads. They worked in such positions "as shakeout, where dust, dirt and sand were cleaned from the molten metal. Coremaking was an even more dangerous and dirty job where many black workers died of gas explosions."[27] Black men also took a large and disproportionate share of the hot and arduous jobs in the coke ovens, where, as labor historian Steven A. Reich notes, "Exposure to extreme heat quickened their heart beat, changed the pitch of their voice, gave them headaches and stomach cramps, and often left them unconscious and in need of hospitalization. . . . Fires burned their clothes, and acid spills scarred their skin."[28] But foundry workers suffered the most profound damage to their health. From a negligible number before 1915, African Americans soon rose to one-third of all foundry workers in the country during and after World War I. They made up over two-thirds of foundry workers in Birmingham, Alabama, and other cities in the South.[29]

African American movement into the industrial workplace coincided with the increasing introduction of "power equipment" in the mines, mills, and factories. These technological innovations increased the amount of dust particles that workers had to breathe and transformed the workplace into a more hazardous environment than before. As one coal miner later recalled, "I have been sick and dizzy off of that smoke many times. . . . That deadly poison is there. . . . It would knock you out too, make you weak as water."[30]

Foundries proved even more deadly for Black workers than the foregoing description of the work would lead us to believe. Silicosis, "a lung disease caused when workers inhale fine particles of silica dust—a mineral that is the primary component of sand, quartz, and granite," took a huge and disproportionate toll on the lives of Black workers in foundry departments across the industrial nation. In their innovative study of silicosis, *Deadly Dust: Silicosis and the On-Going Struggle to Protect Workers' Health*, historians David Rosner and Gerald Markowitz show how it was the introduction of new power machinery, even more so than the dangers of handling molten steel, that created ongoing and relentless inhalation of deadly sand and silica dust that posed the greatest health risk to foundry workers.

Foundry workers even took the deadly minerals home with them. The lethal silica dust "found its way into every crevice or crease in workers' clothing. On their shoes and in their socks. When workers left after a day's toil, they would spit it from their mouths, blow it from their noses, and clear it from their throats—and cough it up from their lungs." Even as the government mandated new health precautions like the wearing of masks, employers of large numbers of Black workers usually ignored such regulations. In 1937, for example, in an Upstate New York foundry, when one Black worker got sick and died from the "deadly dust," according to a pathology report from the Saranac Laboratory, he "was never supplied with masks, ventilating equipment, or the suction devices then being touted as the answer to the industry's silicosis problem."[31]

While the vast majority of women continued to work in the household service sector of the urban industrial economy, they also slowly moved into manufacturing jobs along with Black men. Like their male counterparts, they also occupied the heavy, hot, dirty, and dangerous jobs in much higher proportion than their white counterparts. In New York, a Black female garment worker complained, "Over where I work in the dye factory, they expect more from a colored girl if she is to keep her job. They won't give a colored girl a break." Philadelphia and eastern Pennsylvania glass manufacturers hired Black women workers, presumably because of "their ability to stand the heat without suffering." Women glass workers confronted a hazardous work environment, "where at times bits of broken glass were flying in all directions," exposing them to serious cuts from shards of glass. Cleveland industrialists hired some Black women in the garment industry as "pressers" in accord with the racial stereotype that Black women could "stand heat better than a white girl." Other Black women worked for the wartime railroad industry as "truckers, shearers, and yard workers sorting and hauling scrap and freight."[32]

Southern Black women occupied an even broader range of heavy, hot, and hazardous industrial workplaces than their sisters in the North. In 1919, at Norfolk's Mar-Hof textile company, white men cut fabrics and maintained the machinery, Black men worked as custodians, and white women operated the power machines, inspected finished products, and supervised other women—but Black women occupied "the hot and arduous job of standing over the pressing machines day after day." African American women examined bales of cotton in Houston's cotton compresses and warehouses. They inspected the "dirty or burnt cotton and removed the bad cotton from the bale." In Memphis, Black women took "hot, heavy, dirty," and low-wage jobs in the city's chemical, clothing, and food plants.[33]

Tobacco factories claimed the largest number of Black female industrial workers in Durham, North Carolina. According to historian Leslie Brown, "if there was a job that represented Jim Crow's intent to debase African American women, it was working tobacco."[34] Labor in the tobacco factories duplicated old antebellum practices in many ways. Much like the antebellum system of human bondage in the tobacco industry, the postbellum tobacconists continued to select women workers on the basis of their physical strength and endurance. Brown vividly describes the process of selecting and employing Black women tobacco workers: "Women were selected for positions as though they were on the auction block. On the first day of green season, when the factories began to hire seasonal stemmers, hundreds of Black women gathered in groups at the front steps of the factory. Foremen appeared periodically to select the workers they wanted, choosing the ones who presented the physical characteristics of strength and youth." When queried by an investigator on the employment process, one foreman said, "I rate them by their muscles. . . . The stronger they are the better they are." The destructive impact of tobacco work also paralleled the hazards of the old regime.

The stemming area was a hot, steamy, unventilated room. Black workers toiled with sweat and were covered with dust. Many complained of nausea and coughing, symptoms of respiratory diseases that raced through the factory at epidemic proportions. Their loss of appetite exacerbated malnutrition. African American women suffered horrible working conditions and a number of health risks, evidenced by the regularity of difficult pregnancies, stillbirths, deaths from tuberculosis, and episodes of fainting from heat exhaustion.[35]

In tobacco factories and all along a broad cross-section of urban industrial jobs, Black men and women contracted work-related silicosis, bronchitis, pneumonia, and heart disease, to name a few occupational ailments that they endured.[36] While extractive and manufacturing industries took the greatest toll on the health of Black workers, work regimens in household, domestic, food, and personal service also pressed against the good health of Black workers. The African American Pullman porter, for example, emerged as a widespread symbol of Black men's continued employment in the personal service field. At the height of railroad mileage and passenger travel during the early 1920s, the Pullman Company employed over 9,000 Black porters. These men served some 31 million travelers a year. Another 11,000 mostly African American men worked for other companies on the railroads as coach porters or train porters. Porters remained on call day and night. "If you got any sleep at all," one porter by the name of Leon Long recalled, "that would be in the smoking room. . . . They put on an extra car, so they say I don't get any sleep [for three or four nights]. So I had to set up and do the best I could." The Pullman Company also equipped each coach with a bell to give passengers easy and continuous access to the porter's services.[37]

The health challenges confronting African Americans intensified under the impact of the Great Depression, war, and their aftermath. A series of successive events underscored the precarious health status of African Americans during the interwar and early postwar years. These events included, to name a few, the rise of a debilitating domestic service hiring arrangement called "slave market"; the Hawk's Nest Tunnel construction tragedy in southern West Virginia; the US Public Health Service Tuskegee syphilis study; a dilapidated housing disaster in Philadelphia; and the emergence of lead poisoning as a major health hazard affecting Black families and their children in major cities across the country. Emergence of the so-called slave market on streets across depression-era America had its roots in the depression's devastating impact on Black workers and their families.

Depression, War, and the Early Postwar Years

By 1932, unemployment had increased to nearly 25 percent nationwide, but African Americans faced the brunt of rising joblessness and the desperate search for public or private relief to prevent starvation, sickness, and even death. By 1933, urban African American unemployment had increased to nearly three times the rate of whites in St. Louis, Detroit, Chicago, Los Angeles, and Norfolk. As Black men lost their jobs as the "last hired and first fired," in desperation, some took work in the most toxic environments of the depression-era economy. At the same time, white women increasingly displaced Black women from their stronghold in household work as the depression took its toll on white as well as Black women. Declining employment opportunities for Black women fueled the rise of what became known as the depression-era slave-like hiring of household workers, while Black men took work on some of the most hazardous building and construction projects.

The Infamous "Slave Market" and the Hawk's Nest Tunnel

Scores of African American women congregated on sidewalks of major cities across America. They offered their services to white women who drove up in their cars seeking household help at the lowest possible wages, usually no more than $5 for a week's work—washing clothes, ironing, cooking, scrubbing floors, washing windows, tending children, and the list goes on and on. No region of the country was exempt from the disproportionately painful impact of the depression on the health and well-being of the African American community.[38]

In the coalfields of West Virginia, the Great Depression touched off an intensive intraregional search for work to help make ends meet. Black workers struggled to maintain a footing in the coal mining region, hoping that coal jobs would sooner or later return. Their desperation is vividly captured by the Hawk's Nest Tunnel in Fayette County, West Virginia, described by social and labor historians as "the worst industrial disaster in American history." In 1930, the Union Carbide Corporation commissioned the construction firm of Rinehart and Dennis of Charlottesville, Virginia, to dig the tunnel in order to channel water from the New River to Union Carbide's hydroelectric plant near Gauley Bridge. As local historian Mark Rowh noted, "Construction of the tunnel would mean hundreds of jobs, and many saw it as a godsend. Unfortunately, it would prove the opposite."[39]

Requiring extensive drilling through nearly four miles of deadly silica rock, in some areas approaching 100 percent pure silica, the project claimed the lives of an estimated 500 men by its completion in 1935. African Americans were disproportionately hired for the project, and they were the chief victims. They made up 65 percent of the project's labor force and 75 percent of the inside tunnel crew. Official company reports invariably underestimated the number of casualties on the project; even so, they highlight the disproportionate Black deaths among the work crews. According to P. H. Faulconer, president of Rinehart and Dennis, for example, "In the 30 months from the start of driving to the end of 1932, a total of 65 deaths of all workmen, both outside and inside the tunnel occurred, six white and fifty-nine colored." Although the firm was aware of a wet drilling method that was safer, it selected to use the more efficient but lethal dry drilling process, allowing workers to use water "only when state inspectors were expected at the scene."[40]

Later congressional testimony on the event showed that the company doctor had "systematically misled workers who complained of lung ailments." According to the testimonies before Congress, physicians "were not allowed to tell the men what their trouble was." One doctor from the nearby town of Mt. Hope, West Virginia, admitted that he informed the men that they had "tunnelitis." In the face of repeated denials that they knew about the dangers of the Hawk's Nest Tunnel project, company officials and physicians routinely wore face masks to protect themselves but refused such masks for workers. The Great Depression was not only a time of extensive unemployment. It was also a time of extraordinary exploitation and endangerment of the lives of workers who managed to find jobs in hazardous environments like the Hawk's Nest Tunnel.[41]

The USPHS Tuskegee Syphilis Study

Constraints on access to professional medical education for African Americans unfolded alongside the persistence of unethical experimentation on African American bodies in the interest of science and medicine. The onset of the Great Depression intensified this problem for Black people. It produced one of the most callous race-class medical experiments in the nation's history. Between 1932 and 1972, the US Public Health Service (USPHS) carried out its infamous Tuskegee syphilis study among Black men in Macon County, Alabama. The study selected 399 Black men with advanced syphilis disease, and another 201 men who were syphilis-free as a control group. Specifically, the study aimed to observe the long-run effects of "untreated syphilis in the male Negro."[42] As medical historian Susan M. Reverby makes clear, the USPHS actively kept the men "from many forms of treatment (including penicillin when it became available in the late 1940s)." Moreover, the human subjects of the experiment were never given "a clear diagnosis" of their disease. Instead, the USPHS provided "the watchful eye" of a nurse Eunice Rivers along with regular exams, a diagnostic spinal tap, placebos, tonics, aspirins, free lunches, and burial insurance as inducements for their participation in the experiment.[43] Data on the untreated men would be used as a baseline "to compare it to a retrospective, not prospective, study of white men and women done in Oslo, Norway, earlier in the century when little treatment was available."[44]

Public health officials later emphasized that penicillin (an effective drug treatment for syphilis) was not available until a decade after the study had gotten underway.[45] Thus, in their view, it was misleading to condemn researchers for withholding a viable cure at the outset of the experiment. Even so, at the outset of the study, researchers denied the men access to contemporary drug treatments for the disease (including mercury and the arsenic compounds known as "salvasan") on the premise that these treatments were highly toxic and caused perhaps more "harm for patients than potential benefits."[46] Yet, in 1926, six years ahead of the syphilis study, researchers found that "continuous treatment of *early syphilis* (4 or more courses of an arsenical with interim mercury—at least 21 injections of an arsphenamine) reduced clinical or sero relapse to 21%, as against 89.2% in patients receiving 1 to 8 injections of arsenic."[47] In 1932, the same year that the Tuskegee study got underway, the Cooperative Clinical Studies project, consisting of five university hospital clinics and the USPHS, corroborated the results of the 1926 study.[48]

The advent of penicillin actually alarmed public health researchers who fought hard to justify and continue the project on its initial terms. They took extraordinary steps to keep the men from gaining access to the new medication. During the early postwar years, when knowledge of penicillin spread widely among the African American population, one public health service officer lamented that 33 of the 132 men he examined had received penicillin. Fearing possible termination of the project, he quickly discounted the significance of penicillin treatment for the experimental group, concluding that "economics has prevented the majority of our patients from receiving any consistent daily course of treatment." Raymond V. Vonderlehr, a well-regarded USPHS officer, chimed in with his own expression of "hope that the availability of the antibiotics has not interfered too much with the [validity] this project."[49] On another occasion, Vonderlehr asked a local Macon County, Alabama, health director to urge the draft board to avoid drafting members of the study group. Tell them, he said, "that this study of untreated syphilis [over the lifetime of the men involved] is of great importance from a scientific standpoint. It represents one of the last opportunities [given the escalating demand for "informed consent" protocols] which the science of medicine will have to conduct an investigation of this kind."[50]

Although the notion of a strict "informed consent" requirement for research on human subjects did not emerge among medical professionals until the 1960s, the Tuskegee USPHS study nonetheless violated an earlier informal "moral code" that helped to guide medical experiments on human beings during the period. According to historian Martin Pernick, "even before a patients' rights perspective developed around informed consent there was a sense of the importance of 'truth-telling and consent-seeking' in medical practice in the nineteenth and early twentieth centuries."[51]

But the combined impact of historical dynamics of race, class, and gender placed African Americans outside the informal consensual framework that mitigated the harmful impact of medical experimentation for white subjects. The Black human subjects of the experiment believed that they were being treated for syphilis by a team of competent professional physicians and nurses. Moreover, they did not give their consent even in the informal consensual medical environment of the early twentieth century. In short, the US Public Health Service Tuskegee study was perhaps the most painful episode in twentieth-century medical apartheid. It contained "the elements of a sexually transmitted disease, African Americans [racial bias], coercion and lying by government officials, violation of trust between health-care providers and patients, and fear of experimentation, wrapped into a forty-year narrative [once exposed to the public by the Associated Press in 1972] with multiple media replays."[52]

Recent assessments of the Tuskegee study highlight the failure of the US Public Health Service to honor the US government's principles in developing the Nuremberg Code (1947), a set of human rights pronouncements against unethical medical experimentation on human subjects, a product of the condemnation of Nazi concentration camp experiments on Jews during World War II. According to ethicist Jay Katz, US medical science professionals and public health officials excused their behavior in the Tuskegee case on the premise that the Nuremberg Code was "a code for barbarians and not for civilized physician-investigators." Some thirty years later, one USPHS professional, John R. Heller, underscored this contradiction in US health policy in the Tuskegee case. When historian James H. Jones asked Heller "whether or not the Nuremberg Code had given them pause in the Study, Heller took umbrage at the question and said to Jones, 'But they were Nazis.'"[53]

Involuntary medical experimentation on Black patients did not end with the Tuskegee study but persisted and even intensified during the postwar years. As reproductive rights historian Johanna Schoen makes clear, by the 1950s, social policy professionals and the medical establishment had replaced older "hereditary" racist theories with new "culture of poverty" ideas to justify the forced sterilization of poor women. At the same time, as a consequence of civil rights legislation and movements for racial equality in the medical field, social welfare programs designed to serve poor people brought African Americans "into closer contact with social workers and thus with state-supported sterilization" clinics nationwide. Across the United States, African Americans increased from 31 to 48 percent of all welfare recipients between 1950 and 1961 alone. In North Carolina, to take one state-level example, Black people rose from 23 to 64 percent of all "state-sterilized patients" between the 1930s and the mid-1960s.[54] Various forms of coercion underlay these rising numbers. In his groundbreaking essay on the Montgomery, Alabama, involuntary sterilization federal court case of *Relf v. Weinberger* (1973), law professor Gregory Michael Door illuminated the discriminatory process leading to the involuntary sterilization of young Black women and girls. I quote at length his description of the case here.

On June 13, Mrs. Minnie Relf welcomed two representatives from the Montgomery Community Action Council (MCAC) into her home. According to Mrs. Relf, these social workers told her that they had noticed boys 'hanging around' her daughters, fourteen-year-old Minnie Lee and twelve-year old Mary Alice. Worried that this social interaction would lead to sexual intercourse, the welfare officials escorted Mrs. Relf and the girls to a local hospital and presented Mrs. Relf with a bureaucratic solution: they placed consent forms in front of her. Mrs. Relf's illiteracy rendered her unable to read the forms; her lack of education further confused the officials' explanations. Mrs. Relf believed that signing the forms would authorize the MCAC's family planning clinic to give her daughters "some shots." Her oldest daughter, seventeen-year-old Katie, had been receiving injections of the then-experimental, long-term birth control drug Depo-Provera from the clinic. Assuming that she was enrolling her youngest daughters in the same program, Mrs. Relf made her mark, an uncertain X, on the signature line of each consent form. A nurse then escorted Mrs. Relf home. The next morning, Mary Alice and Minnie did indeed receive shots—of sedatives—after which they were wheeled into an operating room and surgically sterilized. Unbeknownst to Mrs. Relf, she had made her mark on surgical consent forms authorizing the sterilizations. Two weeks later, on June 27, the Southern Poverty Law Center (SPLC) filed a $1 million lawsuit on Relf's behalf, sparking furious protest. Before the year ended, Americans learned that doctors and overzealous social workers had been targeting poor women, and especially poor women of color, in a nationwide epidemic of sterilization.[55]

Experimentation and unethical treatment of poor Black women patients also included the high-profile cases of Henrietta Lacks (1951) and Fannie Lou Hamer (1961). In the case of Henrietta Lacks, a cervical cancer patient at Johns Hopkins University Hospital, the principal physician handling her care discovered that she had cancer cells with unusual properties that made them ideal for cancer research. Upon her death, without the consent of her husband, the university marketed her cells to medical facilities worldwide and helped to advance cancer research that created a new field called "cell-line culture." In the case of civil rights activist Fannie Lou Hamer, the physician charged with removing an apparently benign uterine fibroid tumor took the liberty of removing her entire uterus and rendering her sterile and unable to bear children. Moreover, she only learned of this crime through the gossip grapevine on the Mississippi sharecropping plantation where she and her family worked.[56]

While these high-profile cases gain the lion's share of scholarly and media attention, other lesser known cases would also later fuel the gradual emergence of grassroots Black reproductive rights struggles. For example, the National Black Women's Health Project, formed in 1984 under the leadership of reproductive rights activist Byllye Avery, had its origins in the early 1970s before and after the US Supreme Court legalized abortions in the case of *Roe v. Wade* (1973).[57]

Public health authorities also neglected the safety and health of Black people in dilapidated rental properties across the urban landscape. In December 1936, for example, Philadelphia became the scene of a major tenement house disaster. The collapse of an old building at 517–519 South 15th Street killed nearly a dozen working-class Black women and children and seriously injured as many others. The city's mayor, S. Davis Wilson, expressed his disbelief at the wreckage and carnage. In an interview with reporters, he said, "This is an emergency of public safety. . . . I saw sights yesterday which I would not have believed possible." The liberal Jewish editor of the *Philadelphia Record* declared his hope that this tragedy would sensitize the community to the lives of "thousands of our fellow citizens" whose "home is the place where the sun doesn't shine; the place where they contract tuberculosis; the place where there isn't any running water; the place that may fall down in the dead of night, smothering, burning— 'Home, Sweet Home.'"[58]

Tenants had repeatedly complained about the poor and inadequate upkeep of the building. Just before its collapse, one tenant, Raymond Blackwell, had pleaded with the landlord, Abraham Samson, to repair the building, describing how "the walls on the second floor front room [are] bulging at least a foot and a half [and] the paper in the kitchen [is] falling off and the walls [have] begun to crack." In 1935, the *Philadelphia Tribune* developed a series of articles on housing among Black Philadelphians, emphasizing "the neglect of city inspectors, price-gouging by white landlords, and substandard facilities within which Black Seventh Warders lived." Calling the area "Hell's Acre," the *Tribune* declared the African American housing stock "no accident," but rather "planned slums." By 1940, over 75 percent of all-white homes in Philadelphia met the city's "minimum standards" of sanitation and safety, but only 46 percent of African American dwellings met these standards. According to historian James Wolfinger, by World War II, Philadelphia's Blacks "found themselves boxed in . . . they were forced to live in the city's oldest, most overcrowded areas." Arthur Faucet, an African American activist during the interwar years, made the same point, recalling how Philadelphia had earlier prided itself as the "City of Homes." "Today," he said, "it would be more nearly correct to point to it as the city of slums."[59]

Racial disparities in the American health care system were not limited to the interwar years. They followed Black people into the emerging Cold War era after World War II. Emblematic of the toxic postwar living spaces of Black urbanites was the rapid spread of lead poisoning of young children during the 1950s and 1960s. Beginning gradually during the 1930s, childhood lead poisoning reached epidemic proportions during the post–World War II years. The widespread use of lead-based paints, made by "combining acidized lead with oil," in low-income housing projects and developments became a major source of sickness among Black children. As the paint chips peeled from the walls of "ghetto" housing, young poor children consumed the particles. As one environmental historian explained, "Malnourished children found the paint chips sweet tasting, and poor, overworked . . . parents could not prevent ingestion."

Chips of lead-based paints not only cause "severe illness and occasional death, but also long-term developmental disorders and mental handicaps." During the 1950s and 1960s, lead poisoning reached epidemic proportions in poor Black neighborhoods. Until then, according to Rosner and Markowitz, the lead industry had developed commanding control over scientific research and public knowledge of the issue through its powerful Lead Industry Association and a roster of private research institutes and philanthropic foundations, including Mellon Institute, the Charles F. Kettering Foundation, and the American Public Health Association.[60]

Health inequities were not solely the product of unhealthy and dangerous jobs and living conditions. They were also a product of the persistence of white supremacist ideas and practices in the medical field, ongoing neglect of African American health care needs by policymakers and medical professionals, and continuing subtle and not so subtle assaults on the African American medical infrastructure.

Enduring White Supremacist Ideas in the Medical Field

As discussed previously, some social Darwinists gradually abandoned their beliefs in inherent differences between Black and white bodies and adopted environmentalist perspectives on disease. They expressed increasing consciousness of the ways disease crossed the Jim Crow color line and imperiled the health of both Blacks and whites. But the vast majority of medical experts as well as laypeople continued to embrace racialist definitions of disease as a product of inherited racial differences between African Americans and whites. According to medical historian David McBride, racial interpretations of illness persisted under a rubric he dubbed "anatomic geneticism."[61]

This version of racist medical science built explicitly upon earlier social Darwinist ideas and research findings in such fields as population studies, anatomy, and microbiology. These medical researchers and theorists sought to "identify racial differences within the physiology or biochemical operations of the body and establish new sets of 'physical' criteria for the races based upon a blend of physiology, static genetics, and anthropology." Accordingly, these analysts emphasized the existence of what they saw as distinctive "blood-type groups" to redraw the color line in the era of the Great Migration. These ideas gained sharp expression in the research of sociologists Edward Reuter and human biologist Samuel J. Holmes. In a series of essays leading to his major text, *The Negro's Struggle for Survival* (1937), Holmes focused attention on the health and medical consequences of the massive Great Migration of Southern Blacks into the nation's major cities, concluding that African American migration, despite providing Black people a degree of upward mobility, was most likely a "prelude to [their] extinction."[62]

Throughout World War II and the early postwar years, African Americans complained that the medical profession "seemed unconcerned" about the conditions of their health, especially in the expanding inner-cities of the nation. Declining TB and venereal disease rates nationwide, assisted by the invention of effective new drug treatment protocols, encouraged the mainstream medical establishment to frequently overlook, downplay, or ignore the persistent health crisis around TB, VD, and other diseases within African American urban communities. In a wartime radio broadcast in Charleston, West Virginia, the Black physician Dr. William A. Beck, a professor of medicine at Meharry Medical College, told listeners that TB remained the "second leading cause of death" among Black Americans. As part of the solution to this problem, Beck also called for the elimination of the color line in the nation's medical facilities and equal access to medical care for Black citizens. Similarly, in 1946, on a popular radio show in New York City, the Black physician Dr. George D. Cannon condemned the city and the medical profession for the TB epidemic among Black residents. "Here is a contagious disease killing people," he said, but the mayor, city health officials, and the nation's medical leaders "don't get excited."[63]

Along with the neglect of African American health care needs and unethical experiments on their bodies, across industrial America, established mental health services discriminated against Black patients.[64] To take one prominent example, in its treatment of Black patients, the Georgia state hospital for the mentally ill expanded its program of agricultural production, now increasingly intermixed with convict laborers. During the years between the world wars, the state's mental institution achieved "distinction" as the only state agency with its own slaughter house or "abattoir." According to historian Mab Segrest, "Six pages of the 1950 report detail its work slaughtering 3,346 hogs with a 'live weight' of 649,610 pounds. . . . Workers at the abattoir also slaughtered 2,619 cows, for 2,045,403 pounds of 'live weight' and $320,539.82 of 'live cost.'"[65]

Meanwhile, the state of Georgia also moved into the ranks of the expanding eugenics movement and worked to eliminate the most severely emotionally and physically handicapped among Black patients. In 1918, the state legislature commissioned the National Committee for Mental Hygiene (NCMH), an active proponent of the eugenics movement, to study the feasibility of passing a eugenics law that would permit forced sterilization and even euthanasia for the most disabled members of the patient population. The commission enthusiastically recommended the development of "a farm colony" devoted exclusively to what it described as "mental defectives." Through a series of IQ tests, this population would be divided into two groups: an able-bodied group that would be "usefully and profitably employed" and a second group deemed unfit and presumably candidates for "forced sterilization or euthanasia." In the wake of the NCMH report, the state legislature established a new Georgia Training School for Mental Defectives (also known as the Gracewood State School and Hospital), located in a rural area near Augusta.[66]

Racist medical science and health care policies intersected with discriminatory real estate practices and further undercut the health of Black Americans. As the Great Migration converged with the Great Depression, white property owners doubled and even tripled their revenue by subdividing large single-family homes into single-room, small kitchenette apartments for newcomers.[67] The increasing conversion of single-family homes into rental flats reinforced overcrowding, disease, and unhealthy conditions in Black urban communities. African Americans pressed every conceivable space, including bathtubs and pool tables, into service for sleeping purposes. They took up residence in makeshift bunkhouses, railroad boxcars, boathouses, and shanties in Pittsburgh and the steel towns of western Pennsylvania and elsewhere. Other migrants lived in neighborhoods that abutted outlying rural areas and sometimes "squatted on vacant land," living in tents, shacks, trailers, automobiles, and even "chicken coops" without "running water, electricity, sanitation facilities, paved roads," or garbage collection and streetlights. For some migrants, particularly in cities in the South, these conditions blurred the lines between rural and urban life and labor. A migrant from Greenwood, Mississippi, later recalled moving to Memphis in 1936 and living with her brother in a "shanty." The place was little more than "a shack on a rural plantation."[68]

Poor housing and living conditions reinforced the painful impact of disease on the health and well-being of Black families and their communities. Tuberculosis was the number-one cause of death among African Americans nationally during the industrial age. The TB rate for whites and Blacks in the North and South declined between 1920 and 1933, but the TB rate for Northern Blacks rose between 1923 and 1926 and again between 1929 and 1930. Between roughly 1915 and 1920 alone, Detroit's African American TB deaths increased from about 208 per 1,000 population to 237 per 1,000 people; the white rate went down, from 97 in 1915 and 77 in 1920. A significant racial gap also characterized the city's infant mortality rate—118 deaths per 1,000 births among Blacks compared to 76 per 1,000 among whites.[69]

By the early 1930s, according to the records of physicians, hospitals, and Rosenwald Fund-Public Health Service research, venereal disease, especially syphilis, increasingly overtook TB as "the leading public health crisis" for the nation's Black population.[70] During World War II, moved partly by the country's patriotic imperative to defeat the Nazi powers and rally to the "health defense of the Nation," medical tests for the first 3 million men considered for military service revealed that the incidence of syphilis was ten times greater among Black than prospective white recruits. At the same time that TB continued to decline for the US population from 150 per 100,000 people in 1918 to just 40 per 100,000 in 1945, the disease remained an important health challenge for Black Americans during and following the interwar years. Between 1940 and 1942, TB was the number-one cause of death for Blacks ages 15 to 34.[71]

Changing standards for the practice of medicine also undercut the African American medical infrastructure and reinforced the debilitating impact of neglect. Assaults on the Black health care system had roots in changes that had transpired on the eve of World War I. Under the impact of the influential Flexner Report on the status of medical school training in the United States and Canada, the number of Black medical schools dramatically declined. By 1923, of the fourteen Black medical schools that had emerged in the United States over time, "only Meharry Medical College and Howard University survived." The two schools for Black physician and nurses training stood virtually alone "as the sole sources of medical training for African Americans" between 1910 and the onset of the Modern Black Freedom Movement of the 1960s. Moreover, racial disparities in doctor/patient ratios were an astounding five to six times higher for Blacks than for whites.[72]

Lopsided doctor/patient ratios would also persist into the years after World War II and help to spark the rise of the Modern Black Medical Rights Movement. The Black medical profession increasingly joined African Americans from all walks of life to challenge the Jim Crow order and demolish medical apartheid. Their efforts intensified in the years after World War II, but they had deep roots in the medical struggles of the interwar years.[73] According to historian David McBride, the Great Migration shifted the medical rights struggle from a prevailing emphasis on heavy grassroots community involvement to an increasing reliance on Black medical professionals—mostly physicians and nurses—and their white allies, physicians and nurses, as well as philanthropists and public health officials. As such, emerging medical justice advocates advanced the notion that "institutionalized discrimination [particularly segregation] was the greatest obstacle to black health and medical progress."[74]

Emergence of the Modern Medical Rights Struggle

Industrial-era Blacks launched new and more militant health movements alongside the rise of the "New Negro" phenomenon of World War I and the 1920s. Community-based campaigns to improve the health of Black people spread across urban and rural America. As early as 1915, in the year of his death, Booker T. Washington and the Negro Business League spearheaded the establishment of Negro Health Week. Over the next two decades and beyond, the emergence of a grassroots Black health movement vigorously pressed the US Public Health Service to address health inequities among African Americans, including the widespread incidence of tuberculosis.

Interwar and Early Postwar Era

National Negro Health Week activities engaged a broad cross-section of African American organizations, including the Urban League, NAACP, churches, and Black public health nurses. By the early 1930s, under the increasing impact of the Black health care movement, the federal government took over Negro Health Week activities. With financial support from the Rosenwald Fund, Negro Health Week became "an official," year-round, "government-sponsored black health movement," which soon produced the *National Negro Health News*, a publication of the US Public Health Service.[75]

Nationwide, African American churches and ministers regularly added the health care message of education to Sunday services and sermons. Actively encouraging education on modern medical science and treatments, medical activists found ample opportunity to quote from Hosea 4:6: "My people are destroyed for lack of knowledge." In April 1918, amid the emerging flu pandemic, the Urban League and a host of Black ministers distributed over 20,000 copies of public health literature provided by government agencies. Schoolchildren participated in Negro Health Week parades. The popular Black weekly *Pittsburgh Courier* regularly published a schedule of times and places of health events, including health education parades through different parts of the African American community.[76]

In addition to churches and local branches of the National Urban League, the Black nationalist movement led by Marcus Garvey also addressed the medical challenges posed by the white supremacist medical system. In August 1920, over 25,000 national and international members of the Universal Negro Improvement Association (UNIA) attended the First International Conference of the Negro Peoples of the World at Liberty Hall in New York City. The conference concluded with passage of its famous "Declaration of Rights of the Negro Peoples of the World." This declaration elevated health care for Black people to a central place in the fight for the full liberation of African people. The document boldly denounced medical Jim Crow. "It is an injustice to our people and a serious impediment to the health of the race to deny competent licensed Negro physicians the right to practice in the public hospitals of the communities in which they reside, for no other reason than their race or color." The organization also answered the exclusion of Black nurses from the Red Cross nurses corps by establishing the Black Cross Nurses (BCN). The first BCN unit emerged in Philadelphia during the spring of 1920 and soon spread to UNIA chapters across the country.[77]

In the 1930s, the Black medical profession worked with the radical National Negro Congress (NNC), an umbrella organization closely allied with the new interracial mass production unions in the Congress of Industrial Organizations and members of the US Communist Party. Under the leadership of A. Philip Randolph, head of the all-Black Brotherhood of Sleeping Car Porters, the NNC encompassed a broad cross-section of African American civic, civil rights, social welfare, religious, and political organizations. Early on in its work, in 1936, the NNC counted more physicians than lawyers among its coordinating committee. Moreover, among the organization's six vice presidents, there were two physicians—Charles A. Lewis of Philadelphia and Robert A. Simmons of Massachusetts.

At its national conference in 1937, the NNC devised a strong health agenda. Its health resolution accented the organization's keen consciousness of the "the intimate relation between Health and the Economic and Social welfare of the people." The health resolution not only called for the expansion of hospitals and maternity and child health care for Black people but also pushed for the expansion of unemployment relief to include "food, dental care, eyeglasses, and medicine." It also firmly proposed that Black representatives receive appointment to "the planning committees of all government and private health agencies."[78]

Beginning gradually during the massive March on Washington during the 1940s, the medical rights movement intensified under the impact of the Modern Black Freedom and Black Power movements during the1950s and 1960s. The Modern Black Liberation Movement called for an end to the Jim Crow order across all categories of African American life, including medical apartheid. Initially, however, post–World War II health activists pinned their hopes on the fight for national health insurance. For a brief moment, the NAACP's National Medical Committee, the National Medical Association (NMA), and influential Black physicians like W. Montague Cobb, the Howard University medical school professor, endorsed the campaign for the Wagner-Murray-Dingell national health insurance bill (S1606). National health insurance for the entire nation, they believed, would be the most promising national policy initiative toward improving the health of Black Americans.[79]

In his testimony before congressional hearings on the subject, Montague Cobb underscored the committee's belief that the universal health plan would open up health services "for all of the nation's needy regardless of race or incomes, and at the same time finance the black physician and black hospital network." In his congressional testimony on behalf of the bill, NMA president Dr. E. I. Robinson urged passage of the measure as evidence that the health problems of African Americans were "inextricably tied up with his economic situation rather than with any inherent racial factor." But conservative resistance, led by the American Medical Association and its allies, killed the measure amidst the expanding Cold War and growing fears about the Soviet Union and the "Communist threat" to American democratic institutions. The mainstream medical profession turned increasingly toward "clinical detection and curative treatment" for disease over consideration of the social conditions of Black communities that impacted their health.[80]

Desegregating the Medical Establishment

During the early post–World War II years, the call to desegregate American medical institutions had taken a back seat to the fight for national health insurance, but this movement did not disappear. Following defeat of the national health insurance movement, Black medical and health care activists escalated their engagement with the massive grassroots movements to demolish the segregationist order, including medical apartheid. The 1963

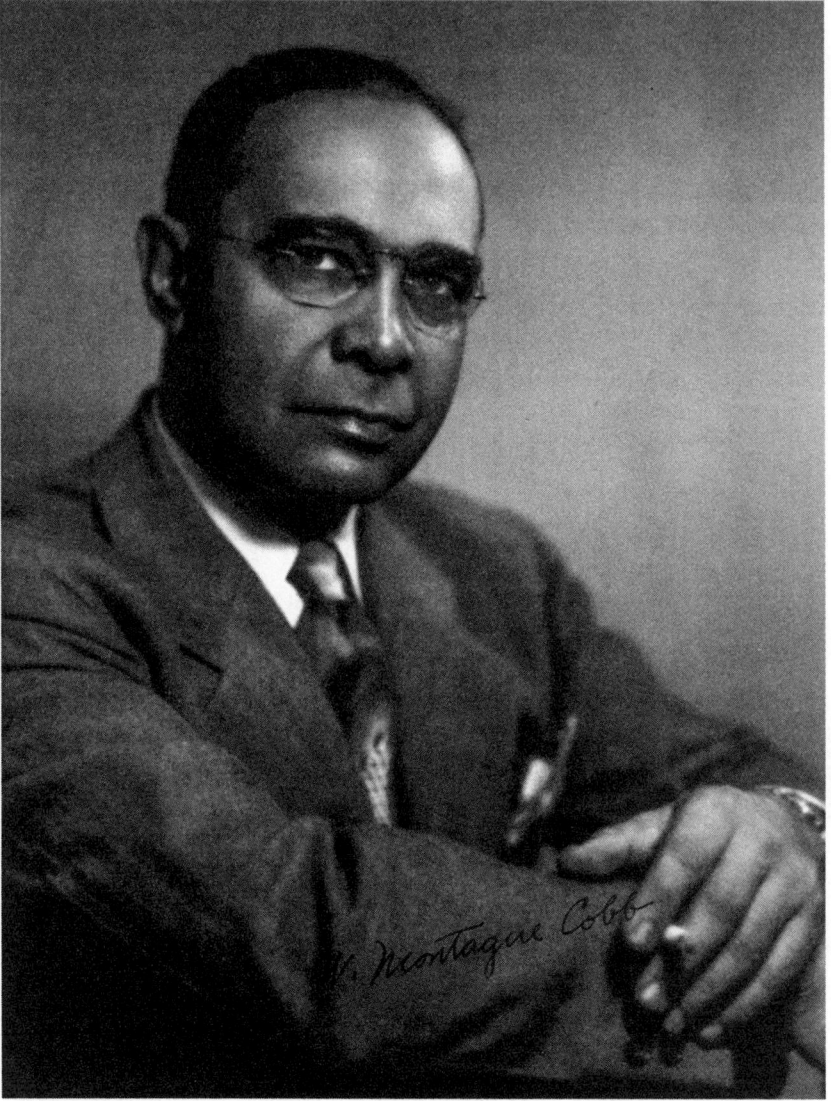

Dr. W. Montague Cobb (1904–90), physician and medical rights activist. Reprinted from H. M. Morais, *The History of the Negro in Medicine* (New York: Publishers Company, 1967), 143.

March on Washington highlighted the increasing convergence of medical and political rights movements within the African American community. President of the NMA, Dr. John A. Kenney Jr., son of the earlier leader of the organization, articulated this fundamental change in posture among Black medical professionals. "The time has come in the problems that confront physicians, especially . . . Negro physicians, that something more than talk is absolutely necessary."[81]

Similarly, as plans for the march took shape, Montague Cobb declared, "For seven years we have invited them [representatives of the American Medical Association and other major hospital organizations] to sit down with us and solve the problem. . . . By their refusal to confer they force action by crisis. And now events have passed beyond them. The initiative offered is no longer theirs to accept." At its 1963 national convention, the National Medical Association passed its historic "Resolution in Support of Mass Protests Against Racial Discrimination." This resolution opened the door for Black medical professionals to join the expanding protests against white supremacy in all walks of life, including the health care system.[82]

The medical rights movement expanded under the leadership of the NMA and the Medical Committee for Civil Rights, an interracial medical rights organization, formed in 1964. The health activism of these organizations increasingly converged with the health care initiatives and programs of the NAACP, NUL (National Urban League), and SCLC (Southern Christian Leadership Conference). The medical needs of the nonviolent direct action protesters soon precipitated the development of their own grassroots medical services. In New York City, the Medical Committee for Civil Rights, later the Medical Committee for Human Rights (MCHR), established health clinics to treat activists under attack on the front lines of the struggle for Modern Black Freedom. Beginning with a focus on the needs of activists, the civil/human rights health clinics soon discovered the immense day-to-day health challenges facing poor and working-class Black communities across the South. They gradually incorporated local residents into their network of health services and dispatched over a hundred volunteers to Mississippi during the Mississippi Summer Project.[83] Widely known as the "medical arm of the civil rights movement," MCHR activism peaked during the early 1970s. Thereafter, it shifted focus to the New Left anti-Vietnam movement and gradually declined.[84]

Under the growing impact of the nonviolent direct action phase of the civil rights movement, the Civil Rights Acts of 1957, 1960, 1964, and 1965 gradually demolished the Jim Crow system. Although the most significant changes occurred in the legislature, the slow methodical use of the law and the courts also produced results that undermined the old order. The medical dimensions of the civil rights movement culminated in the US Supreme Court case of *Simkins v. Moses H. Cone Memorial Hospital* (1963). Spearheaded by a group of Black physicians, nurses, and patients in Greensboro, North Carolina, this case successfully challenged segregation and racial discrimination in medical institutions funded by the state. The medical desegregation movement would pick up steam in the 1960s, but it had deep roots in the interwar years with the desegregation of Harlem Hospital in New York City, for example. By the mid-1930s, African Americans had organized a grassroots medical movement that resulted in the employment of rising numbers of Black physicians and interns from both predominantly white and Black medical schools. As historian Adam Biggs notes in his study of the institutional desegregation of Harlem Hospital, medical professionals trained on different sides of the color line, both claiming the militant mantle of the "New Negro," soon clashed over competing visions for the future of the institution.[85]

By the mid-1960s, in addition to dismantling the legal segregation of Blacks and whites in the nation's medical system, the medical rights movement had also created a vibrant federally funded network of neighborhood health centers (NHCs) under President Lyndon Baines Johnson's War on Poverty program. At decade's end, the Office of Economic Opportunity (OEO) had funded over a hundred NHCs nationwide. US Department of Health, Education, and Welfare (HEW) funded another fifty of these centers and gradually expanded the access of poor Black families to professional medical care. In 1965, against stiff AMA opposition, African Americans and their white allies also gained a major victory with passage of Medicare and Medicaid legislation, increasing federal support for the health care of poor and working-class families. Medical historians credit the NMA with this victory over the Jim Crow medical profession.[86]

As the Jim Crow medical order collapsed under the growing weight of the Modern Black Freedom Struggle and the passage of new civil rights legislation, activists deepened rather than eased their push for grassroots solutions to the health dilemmas confronting poor and working-class Black communities. Grassroots Black medical activism gained even greater and more militant expression in movements to wipe out lead poisoning in poor and working-class Black urban neighborhoods; the rise of the Black Panther Party and its free health clinics; and local innovative health care initiatives like the creation of free ambulance services. Under the leadership of Ivory

Perry, son of an Arkansas sharecropper, and Wilbur Thomas, a young African American scientist, a grassroots phalanx of African American community organizations—churches, schools, and a plethora of war on poverty social service workers and organizations—staged a massive assault on the lead poisoning issue in St. Louis, Missouri.

In 1970, their efforts resulted in the formation of an ad hoc organization called the People's Coalition Against Lead Poisoning. The People's Coalition fought for and secured the city's first municipal ordinance mandating testing of children for lead poisoning, thereby acknowledging the problem as more widespread than heretofore admitted by public health officials and policymakers. By 1971, the St. Louis campaign against lead poisoning had transformed the phenomenon from an obscure place on the Black urban landscape into a citywide issue with profound implications for Black urban communities nationwide. As environmental historian Robert R. Gioielli concludes, "Knowledge that all children were at risk to be poisoned or suffer a variety of unknown mental problems, was what fed lead poisoning activism in St. Louis and similar protests in cities across the country."[87]

Formed in 1966, the Black Panther Party soon launched its People's Free Medical Centers (PFMCs). Local party members forged bonds with both "lay and *trusted-expert*" doctors, nurses, and students in training for the health professions. These volunteers provided free "basic preventive care, diagnostic testing," dentistry, and referrals to other appropriate medical facilities for specialized treatment. Grassroots community-based activists also established the Black Panther Party's ambulance service in Winston-Salem, North Carolina, and Freedom House Ambulance Service in Pittsburgh. In the Steel City, authorities initially placed emergency ambulance services in the police department, a decision that placed the city's Black poor at a severe and even deadly disadvantage. In 1968, to counter the city's discriminatory emergency health service for the city's historic Hill District community, activists launched the Freedom House Ambulance Service. Funded by the Maurice Falk Medical Fund, under the leadership of director Philip Hallen, Freedom House Ambulance Service set out to train a core of community-based emergency workers that many believed were "untrainable."[88]

Through the services of Dr. Peter Safar of Presbyterian University Hospital, these workers gained training in the techniques of "emergency care in the streets." About 50 percent of the initial Freedom House recruits had not completed their high school education before entering training for emergency medical care, but a carefully trained corps of community-based

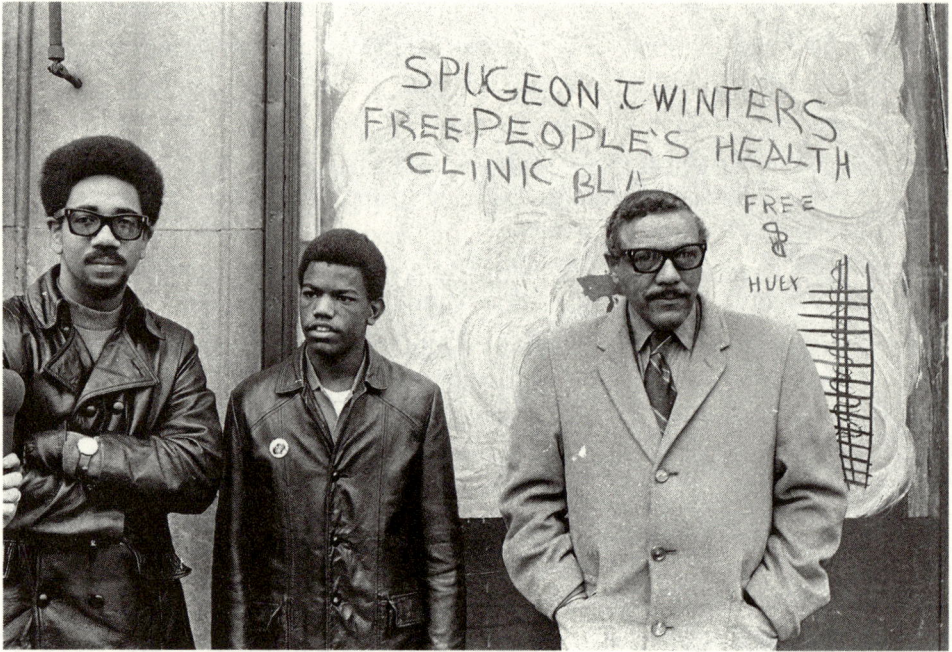

Spurgeon Jake Winters Free People's Health Clinic, Chicago. A photo of the dedication of the clinic shows Illinois Black Panther Party chapter founder (and future politician) Bobby Rush (*left*) with two unidentified men. The clinic's namesake had died in a shootout with police a month earlier. Courtesy of Chicago History Museum/Carnegie Museum of Art, via Getty Images.

emergency workers soon entered the field and helped to mitigate suffering and save lives. A comparative study of police versus Freedom House services revealed that only 11 percent of Freedom House cases involved improper treatment compared to 62 percent of police cases. White residents seeking ambulance service sometime asked the dispatcher to "send Freedom House." In 1975, the city of Pittsburgh terminated its contract with Freedom House and established its own emergency medical services (EMS). But the city's grassroots Black health care movement had not only helped to save African American lives; it had also pioneered a form of medical service that would spread nationwide during the late twentieth century.[89]

Persistence of the Race- and Class-Divided Medical System

In fundamental ways, termination of the Freedom House Ambulance Service also underscored the persistence of the nation's class and racially segmented medical system, even as the desegregation of medical institutions proceeded apace. Well into the 1960s, the nation's medical system maintained most of its market-driven characteristics along with "its structure of race- and class-based inequities, and its middle-class leadership, ideology, and orientation." Under the impact of massive federal funding under the Hill-Burton Act of 1947, all aspects of the US health care system dramatically expanded. The medical field became the nation's third largest industry "in terms of manpower, with a workforce of 2.5 million people and a significant portion of the nation's economy." Between 1947 and 1971, the medical profession received $3.7 billion in federal funds, matched by another $9.1 billion of private funding. Together, these resources resulted in the rise of academic health centers (AHCs) that emphasized "prestige, research, and training instead of delivering primary health services to needy populations."[90]

The AHCs reinforced class and racially stratified and unequal health care across urban America. While Blacks gained increasing access to these large urban public hospitals, the quality of care suffered as the AHCs prioritized research and education over careful patient care. Large predominantly Black urban poor and "public aid populations" were treated as "training material" for major medical schools and research institutions. In their report for the Health Policy Advisory Center (Health-PAC), Barbara and John Ehrenreich called attention to this debilitating phenomenon in big city hospitals: "As interns and residents, young doctors get their training by practicing on the hospital ward and clinic patients—generally non-white. Later they make their money by practicing for a paying clientele—generally white. White patients are 'customers'; black patients are 'teaching materials.' White patients pay for care with their money, black patients pay with their dignity and comfort."[91]

Intertwined with the continuation of class and racially divided health care, African Americans confronted a persistent strain of white supremacist medical ideas and practices. The Black medical profession waged spirited struggles against remaining racist underpinnings of medical science and health care practices in the United States. Although they were encouraged by the emergence of a wider cohort of supportive anti-racist white colleagues during the interwar years, they did not relent in advancing their own challenges to social Darwinist conceptions of race and health care in the nation's mainstream medical profession. An expanding list of innovative Black medical professionals contested the refurbished forms of racist medical beliefs that emerged during the interwar years.

African American critics of racialist interpretations of disease and African American health care included Louis Wright, a New York surgeon and member of the NAACP's national board; T. K. Rawless, a dermatologist; Dr. Charles Drew; and H. L. Harris, a Chicago-based physician and public health researcher, among many others. In 1926, when Frederick L. Hoffman reiterated conclusions reached in his earlier racist portrait of African American urban life, Black medical professionals, most notably H. L. Harris, swiftly countered Hoffman's new research but ultimately old perspectives on African American health and prospects for the future.[92]

A few years later, as the Great Depression got underway, Louis Wright reviewed Samuel J. Holmes's *The Negro's Struggle for Survival*. He roundly criticized Holmes for misusing evidence to make his case for Black inferiority. As an accomplished surgeon who had operated on many Black and white bodies, Wright was especially incensed by Holmes's claim that "the skin of the negro was thicker than the skin of white people." Wright declared that "all races vary in the degree of thickness of their skins, and even individuals *within* the same race do likewise."[93] Unlike Hoffman, however, Holmes seemed to give in to some of the withering criticism leveled against his work on African Americans. Writing in the *Journal of Negro Education* in 1937 on the causes of high African American mortality rates from disease, he remarked, "That the Negro is 'constitutionally inferior' to the whites, as was formerly asserted by some writers, is a conclusion devoid of adequate foundation. With the possible exception of his greater proneness to tuberculosis and the acute respiratory infections, he is, on the whole, probably a better animal than the white man." But he swiftly pivoted back around to his original racial conception of disease, concluding that "granting that the higher mortality of the Negro from most diseases is due to an unfavorable economic and educational status, these diseases are nevertheless selective as a result of inherited racial peculiarities."[94]

Into the 1950s, African Americans and their anti-racist white supporters crafted research projects that aimed not only to document the status of African American health care but also strike blows at continuing remnants of social Darwinist thinking in the medical profession. Emblematic of these studies was a mid-1950s study by the Committee to End Discrimination in Chicago Medical Institutions. Titled "What Color Are Your Germs?," this study reported some sixty-five hospitals and 6,000 doctors serving the medical needs of the city, but nearly 50 percent of all Blacks received medical attention at one facility—Cook County Hospital. Clearly, the medical profession hoped to limit African American access to mainstream hospitals and private physician practices.[95]

Clash and Accommodation of "Folk" and Professional Medicine

At the same time that African Americans fought against discriminatory medical ideas and health policies, they also continued their attacks on traditional medical remedies among poor and working-class Black families. The persistence of such folk beliefs, they firmly believed, impeded the delivery of modern and more effective treatments for Black patients. African American medical professionals and their white allies lamented the failure of large numbers of poor and working-class Blacks to embrace modern medical innovations and treatment for various diseases. In 1926, for example, the National Urban League published the results of a survey, "Superstition and Health," designed to help stamp out what it dubbed misleading and dangerous folk medicine, holdovers from African American life under slavery and later Jim Crow. Defining migrant medical beliefs as "cherished superstitions and false knowledge," one young Black physician described how such beliefs "govern Negroes in illnesses and hamper recoveries" prescribed by modern medical science and practice.

The young doctor further concluded that this "fatalism exasperates the physician, for it ties his hands and tends to nullify his efforts." Hence, the National Urban League, the Black medical profession, and educated Black social welfare workers considered "breaking through the indigenous health system of the Black working class" as a vital priority in their efforts to improve the health and well-being of African American families and communities. By the beginning of World War II, the Tuskegee Institute offered professional training for small numbers of midwives, designed to reduce the pool of informally trained but popular traditional midwives.[96]

Nonetheless, into the 1930s and beyond, the African American folk health system retained a powerful hold on the urban Black working class—North, South, and West. One Black physician, Peyton F. Anderson, president of the Central Harlem Medical Society, described traditional Black healers of the twentieth century as "parasites" and "a curse upon our group." He vigorously urged a declaration of war against them. Despite these hostile professional assaults on the old medical ways, they remained deeply embedded in African American religious culture and beliefs that "health was part of a total protection provided by God." Hence, large numbers of African Americans continued to place their "faith" in "faith" healers and, especially, midwives for the delivery of their babies over professionally trained physicians. In 1937,

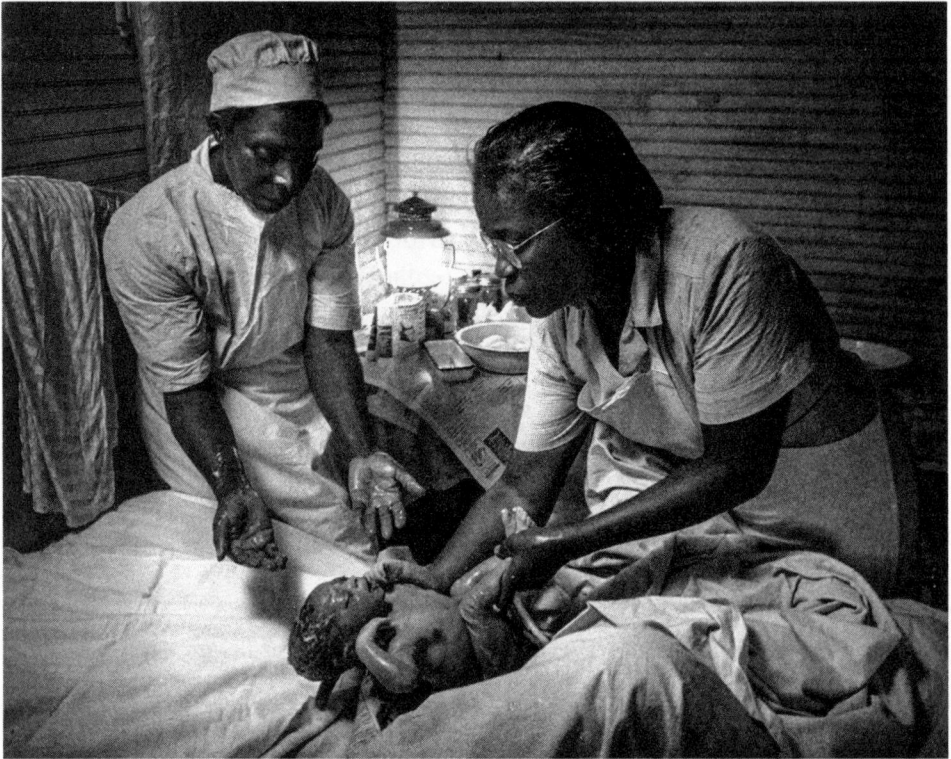

Maude Callen, nurse-midwife, who served rural Black communities in North Carolina during the 1940s and 1950s. W. Eugene Smith, American (1918–78), *Maude Callen with Newborn Baby*, 1951. Gelatin silver print, 10 ½ × 13 ⅜ in. The Nelson-Atkins Museum of Art, Kansas City, Missouri. Gift of Hallmark Cards, Inc., 2005.27.4360. © The Heirs of W. Eugene Smith. Courtesy of Nelson-Atkins Digital Production and Preservation.

for example, midwives continued to deliver over 50 percent of newborn infants in the rural South and over a quarter of all Black babies born in the urban North and South. Even as their access to mainstream medical institutions increased, large numbers of poor and working-class Blacks retained measures of faith in the old ways.[97]

During the mid-1950s, sociologist and civil rights activist Charles S. Johnson lamented "the overbearing power of folk health practices throughout black communities." Some thirty years later, in 1981, professional nurse turned midwife Linda Janet Holmes interviewed a dwindling cohort of African American midwives across the state of Alabama. In her interviews with the women, they often described Black midwifery practices as "winding down," but such practices remained alive in the memory of scores of Black mothers who could recall "the care they received from Black midwives in their communities."[98]

The vast majority of Black medical professionals believed that the ongoing power of traditional medical beliefs and practices partly explained the reluctance of so many African Americans to seek medical help only in times of crisis or life-threatening illness. In order to best serve the entire range of health needs within the African American community, however, the modern Black medical profession would need a deeper and more historical understanding of the complexities of the African American engagement with disease and efforts to find effective cures even as the old Jim Crow order slowly passed away.[99]

Conclusion

The industrial age produced some of the most hopeful and disappointing moments in African American social, political, and medical history. Under the impact of the Great Migration, African Americans made the transition from the nation's most rural to its most urban population. They were no longer primarily a Southern people but a national population, spread across the urban North, South, and West. Their labor helped to fuel the nation's industrial machine, but unlike their white counterparts, they worked under segregated and unequal conditions that proved exceedingly hazardous to their health and well-being. Racial employment policies and social practices confined Black workers to the most dangerous, arduous, low-paying, and health-threatening industrial occupations. Moreover, African American workers and their families inhabited the most dilapidated and unhealthy segments of the urban housing market that made them more vulnerable to respiratory and other disorders than white workers.

As solid as the color line may have been, inequality was not equally shared by all African Americans. Class and gender as well as racial dynamics influenced the health and medical experiences of Black people. As urban historian Earl Lewis declared over three decades ago, "Whereas middle-class blacks found living conditions a discomfort, working-class blacks found them deadly."[100] Across industrial America, African Americans reported a small upper-class "intelligentsia," a "fair sized" middle class, and a massive "proletarian class." Proletarian Blacks lived and worked at the bottom, close to the "bread line." They faced the sharpest and most lethal edges of the urban disease environments.[101]

Even so, starting slowly during the interwar years, industrial-era Black communities nonetheless came together, mobilized their resources, and challenged entrenched patterns of racial and class inequality that undermined the health and well-being of their families and their communities. Their social and political struggles reinforced the rise of the Modern Black Medical Rights Movement that demolished the old Jim Crow health system. But this achievement would not fully hold. Before Black people could genuinely celebrate the passing of the segregationist system, the collapse of the manufacturing economy ushered in a new postindustrial age and the rise of new forms of health inequality along the color line, most notably AIDS, the coronavirus, and the devastation of Hurricane Katrina.

CHAPTER FOUR

Digital Age

Introduction

The old rhetoric of Black biological inferiority and a *propensity* for disease lost favor as the country ended the era of Jim Crow, but new countermeasures by white opponents of Black advancement required new strategies and tactics from those committed to securing medical advances for African Americans. The Modern Black Freedom Movement, in fact, demolished medical apartheid and opened the door for rising numbers of African Americans to move into the mainstream of the nation's health care system as employees, practitioners, and patients. But this process was soon undermined by several developments: the collapse of the manufacturing economy; the growth of new low-wage, service-sector employment with little job security or health insurance benefits, let alone pensions; and hostile conservative attacks on affirmative action programs in medicine as well as employment, housing, and education. In addition to powerful grassroots white opposition to the social welfare state and its services to poor and working-class Black Americans, environmental disasters such as Hurricane Katrina, the ravages of the AIDS epidemic, and the coronavirus pandemic exposed the fault lines of vulnerability. In the face of such challenges and stiff resistance to their struggle for equality, Black urban communities nonetheless built upon their prior industrial-era legacy of medical struggles; strengthened their historically Black health care infrastructure; and forged new strategies to address the demands of the emerging postindustrial age.

The New Service Economy, Health, Class, Ethnic, and Race Relations

Digital age African American work, health, and living conditions unfolded within the larger context of institutional desegregation, the rise of a new service economy, and the ongoing class and racial stratification of the health care system. The fall of the industrial economy emerged at the core of these social transformations in the nation's economy, health, and well-being during the late twentieth and early twenty-first century. Deindustrialization had deep roots in the years after World War II but accelerated and played out during the final decades of the twentieth century. Plant closings and layoffs dominated headline news on the health and welfare of the city, state, and nation. The steel, meatpacking, automobile, and other mass production industries laid off greater numbers of workers, both Black and white, but Black workers bore the brunt of these layoffs. The percentage of Black workers employed in manufacturing jobs steadily declined from about 24 percent in 1979 to under 10 percent in 2007; the white workforce also declined but somewhat less precipitously than African Americans.[1]

While the numbers differed by city, the directionality was constant. The proportion of jobs in inner-city Detroit decreased from nearly 60 percent of all metropolitan area employment during the 1970s to only 21 percent by 1990. In the brief period between 1978 and 1981, a cluster of eight companies accounted for the loss of 18,000 jobs in Los Angeles. Similar to steel and other mass production industries employing large numbers of Black workers, the predominantly Southern textile industry lost over 500,000 jobs between 1980 and 1994. Thousands of Black workers lost jobs in the wake of the textile industry's collapse. Black workers dropped from a peak of about 25 percent of the workforce in 1980 to just over 10 percent as the new century got underway.[2]

As manufacturing jobs steadily slipped away, rising levels of technological unemployment and the gradual movement of former industrial workers and their children into low-wage jobs in the service sector posed new health challenges for digital age Black workers, their families, and their communities. Large numbers of veteran Black industrial workers took jobs in the new low-wage service sector of the deindustrializing economy with few or no benefits or medical coverage. In Gary, Indiana, in 1985, then-mayor Richard Hatcher and a host of other city officials celebrated the opening of a new Wendy's fast-food restaurant as the beginning of new employment opportunities for unemployed steelworkers and their families. Former steelworkers took a share of the eighty new jobs offered by the chain. Wendy's employees earned only $3.35 per hour compared to previous earnings of $15 to $20 per hour, plus benefits, in the unionized steel industry.[3]

Nationwide, by the close of the twentieth century, African Americans and Latino workers occupied an estimated 75 percent of all new jobs created at the bottom 10 percent of the workforce in wages paid, while white workers occupied the same proportion of new jobs created at the top 20 percent of wage levels. Black workers occupied such service jobs as nursing home aides, hospital orderlies, office custodians, hotel maids, and household workers, to name a few. The vast majority of new jobs among African Americans not only paid the lowest wages but offered few if any retirement plans or other forms of economic security. Moreover, such jobs were often temporary or part-time with "unpredictable and unstable hours," few opportunities for promotion, and no labor union representation and protection against workplace injustices. The number of all Black workers in unions plummeted more steeply for Blacks than for white workers, from an estimated 32 to 16 percent between 1983 and 2007.[4] According to sociologist William J. Wilson, US policymakers sanctioned urban poverty by tolerating the reduction of benefits, the rise of involuntary part-time employment, and adjusted for inflation, the decline in the minimum wage to 26 percent lower than its average level during the 1970s. In 1990, a study of urban inequality in four major US cities revealed the highest poverty rate (33 percent) among African Americans in Detroit, compared to 20 percent in Los Angeles, Boston, and Atlanta.[5]

Alongside precarious employment opportunities, conservative social movements also rolled back key gains of the Modern Black Freedom Movement and further undermined the health and well-being of the postindustrial Black urban community, making it more vulnerable to epidemics, pandemics, and other health disasters as compared with white communities.[6] California and Wisconsin emerged at the epicenter of assaults on government benefits for poor and working-class families. In California, white workers and middle-class property owners joined forces and passed Proposition 13 in 1978 and Proposition 209, known as California's Civil Rights Initiative, in 1996. Proposition 13 cut property taxes and severely curtailed the state's capacity to deliver much-needed social services, including health care, to the poor. For its part, Proposition 209 prohibited affirmative action programs from the civil rights era designed to redress historic patterns of discrimination against African Americans, other people of color, and women in public education, employment, and government contracts. Likewise, the Wisconsin plan, dubbed "W-2," tied public assistance programs to a rigorous work requirement that ignored barriers to less educated poor and working people securing adequate wages to provide for their families. Together, the state-level social welfare programs of California and Wisconsin helped to set the pace for the nation. Both anti-welfare and anti–affirmative action movements culminated in the passage of President William Jefferson Clinton's austere and Republican-inspired federal Personal Responsibility and Work Opportunity Reconciliation Act (1996) to end social service programs from the New Deal and civil rights era—as Clinton put it, "to end welfare as we know it."[7]

Navigating the Shrinking Social Service System

The deleterious impact of the new and harsher social welfare policies were not spread evenly across the African American community. Poor and working-class Blacks found it more difficult to navigate these changes than their better educated and wealthier middle- and upper-class counterparts. They lived in what sociologist William J. Wilson dubbed "concentrated urban poverty" and his colleagues Douglas Massey and Nancy Denton labeled "hypersegregation." In a large, delimited area on Chicago's Southside, an estimated 151,000 people, mainly the "nonpoor black middle and working classes," departed these communities during the decade between 1970 and 1980, leaving behind a much more highly concentrated impoverished [and disproportionately unhealthy] black population."[8]

At the same time, new legal mechanisms such as mandatory sentencing for certain offenses, particularly those involving the possession, use, and sale of drugs, allowed national, state, and local authorities to arrest, convict, and incarcerate increasing numbers of young Black men and some women between the ages of 18 and 30. Because of the criminalization of a host of heretofore minor or noncriminal acts, these inmates were sentenced and assigned to work in prison industries for the benefit of the state. During the final two years of the 1990s alone, New York State's Division of Correctional Industries (Corcraft) produced $70 million in income using disfranchised prison labor, reminiscent to some extent of the post-emancipation years of the nineteenth century.[9]

During the final two decades of the twentieth century, as the harsh new carceral and social welfare regimes took hold, drug addiction, crack cocaine, youth violence, and day-to-day forms of police brutality escalated. These painful social trends underscored the many ways that African Americans absorbed the brunt of human suffering under the nation's new antisocial welfare order. Philadelphia's welfare rights activist Roxanne Jones protested the welfare cuts as "human genocide," coming as they did on the heels of the "cold winter we went through, people freezing to death, and not having enough money to pay their fuel bills."[10]

When Lamar, one client of Wisconsin's new program, received his monthly allotment of $628, he paid $550 for rent and had only $78 (about $2.19 cents per day) left over for other necessities. In January 2008, a Milwaukee mother and her two sons were evicted on a cold winter day and forced to move into a homeless shelter, euphemistically called the "Lodge" by area residents. Arleen and her boys joined one in about every eight families nationwide who were unable to pay rent and faced imminent evictions and exposure to the elements. As sociologist Matthew Desmond notes, the rising chorus of evictions took a huge toll on the health and well-being of poor families. Eviction, he said, "invites depression and illness, compels families to move into degrading housing in dangerous neighborhoods, uproots communities, and harms children."[11]

By contrast, highly educated and wealthier middle- and upper-class Blacks benefited from gradual access to better jobs, housing, and health insurance. In the early wake of the Modern Black Freedom Movement, increasing numbers of Black men and women moved up into middle-class occupations. African Americans earning college degrees rose from no more than about 1 percent during World War II and its early aftermath to 10 percent by 2000. A significant portion of these young college-educated Black men and women enrolled in graduate studies and earned advance degrees in such diverse fields as law, medicine, business, finance, science, and engineering as well as the humanities and social sciences. The percentage of African Americans claiming middle-class incomes rose from about 13 percent during the 1960s to 58 percent as the new century got underway. At the same time, better off African Americans gradually moved into more livable, safe, and healthy housing and neighborhoods in outlying areas within the cities as well as in suburbs of major metropolitan regions. Black suburbanization rose during the final three decades of the twentieth century from 15 to 35 percent.[12]

Better educated and wealthier middle-class and upper-class Blacks were by no means immune to the destructive impact of deindustrialization. They were also an internally diverse group with varying levels of resources at their disposal to help guard against hard times. In his groundbreaking study of late twentieth-century Oakland, California, sociologist Eric Brown persuasively argues that the new constraints of the postindustrial political economy fragmented the Black middle class, including health care professionals, into two groups. One group gained employment in predominantly white and more lucrative mainstream institutions, while a second group became self-employed or community-based practitioners serving a predominantly poor and working-class clientele.[13]

Most important, however, the economic recession of 2008 wiped out the homeownership and modest wealth-building gains of large numbers of Black people. An estimated 11 percent of Blacks and 7 percent of whites lost their homes to foreclosures between roughly 2008 and 2012. They were the chief victims of what historian Keeanga-Yamahtta Taylor describes as "predatory inclusion" in the nation's real estate and housing market. As historian

Jacqueline Jones so aptly put it, "Now, instead of denying mortgages to black credit-seekers whether or not they were qualified, banks aggressively marketed toxic financial products to blacks regardless of their financial condition. . . . Indeed, middle class blacks received subprime loans at a rate three times higher than their white counterparts; such loans forced borrowers to pay exorbitantly high fees, interest rates, and hidden and deferred costs."[14]

Between 2005 and 2009, with the vast majority of their wealth invested in homeownership, the median wealth of Black households declined by 53 percent (about $12,000 to $6,000) compared to 16 percent for white households (about $135,000 to $113,000). White households reported retirement funds, pension accounts, and stocks among other sources of wealth besides homeownership. Their wealth also cushioned them against unexpected crises, particularly involving health care, while increasing numbers of Black families lived on the perilous edge of the nation's medical system that was class and still racially divided.[15]

Across the postindustrial landscape, there was a parallel movement of middle-class and affluent whites and some professional-class Blacks from the suburbs, now in decline, to the central cities where property values had plummeted within African American neighborhoods in the wake of violent property riots during the 1960s. These young urban professionals (Yuppies, as they were called at that time) claimed large areas of living space in renovated Victorian homes, previously occupied by poor and working-class Blacks in the central cities. The continuing demolition of old neighborhoods, and the failure to readily rebuild areas burned out by the urban revolts of the 1960s, drove this process of "gentrification" that allowed whites to reclaim prime urban real estate, drive up costs, and force increasing numbers of the Black poor and working class to disperse to other poor areas of the city, leave for the South, or migrate to deteriorating sections of white working-class or lower-middle-class suburbs on the periphery of cities as diverse as Harlem, Boston, San Francisco, Philadelphia, Savannah, Charleston, and Baltimore. In Charleston, young urban professionals and businesspeople converted former slave quarters into expensive apartments. In Washington, DC, alley dwellings formerly occupied by the city's poorest residents now housed US senators and congressional members, among other urban elites.[16]

During the 1970s, after nearly a century of steady movement out of the rural South, the tide of Black population movement turned southward again. Rather than returning to the rural South, however, most returnees and their children and grandchildren from the North and West moved to the expanding urban South. As historian Ira Berlin notes in his epic synthesis of Black population movements, the new Southern migrants and returnees worked in offices, shops, and factories of the urban South and "navigated the streets and alleys of the inner city."[17] Simultaneously, the movement of African and Caribbean immigrants into cities in the North and West offset somewhat the reverse migration of Black people to the South. By the end of the twentieth century, an estimated 1.3 million people of African descent had entered the United States. As the new century got underway, nearly one-tenth of the African American population was "an immigrant or the child of an immigrant." In New York, immigrants and their children made up over 50 percent of the total Black population. The new immigrants and their children gradually transformed the ethnic composition of Black urban communities and their class structures. They also shared with their American-born counterparts rising levels of incarceration, lethal police violence, and recurring assaults on their physical and emotional well-being. In 1999, to take a prominent example, New York City police officers murdered the unarmed West African student Amadou Diallo. In the aftermath of Diallo's murder, Manthia Diawara, a New York University professor of African descent, declared that the African in America "bears the curse of Cain." "In America they, too, are considered black men, not Fulanis, Mandingos, or Wolofs."[18]

Emergence of the digital age dramatically transformed the context of African American medical history, health care, and the larger fight for medical as well as economic, political, civil, and human rights. As the new service economy gained ground, the social welfare state lost ground. The old manufacturing economy nearly disappeared, while the postindustrial era of immigration brought a variety of new people into the city. Rising numbers of African, Caribbean, and American-born Black and white gentrifiers moved into heretofore predominantly Black urban spaces and neighborhoods. These shifting socioeconomic and demographic processes continue to unfold today, with profound implications for the current status of Black health and the ongoing fight to demolish a medical system that is racially and class stratified.

Limits of the Modern Medical Rights Movement

The cresting of the medical rights movement during the civil rights era converged with the increasing collapse of the industrial economy. Black men and women as well as immigrants of African descent shared in the opening up of greater opportunities in the medical profession during the late 1960s and early 1970s. By 1980, for example, Black women physicians had increased to 25 percent of all Black physicians and to nearly 33 percent a decade later. At the same time, immigrants of color augmented the ranks of American-born Black doctors. Black physicians from Africa and the Caribbean increased from negligible numbers at the outset of the period to about 25 percent of the nation's Black women doctors and about "one-fifth of the nation's doctors overall." The lion's share of these Black medical professionals "clustered mainly in the primary care specialties," including family group practice, pediatrics, or general internal medicine, serving predominantly poor and working-class Black clients.[19]

The heralded achievements of the civil rights movement confronted a swift and powerful setback during the final decades of the twentieth century. As early as 1976, at the Atlanta University conference on Black health care, Dr. J. Alfred Cannon described how the emerging post–civil rights era Black community faced a growing health care crisis. In his words, the era of high African American national and international "visibility, relevance and significance" was fast coming to an end. In his view, the progress made against medical apartheid was insufficient and remaining disparities threatened to undermine *the very survival of black America."* In 1983, Margaret M. Heckler, secretary of the Department of Health and Human Services (DHHS), established the Secretary Task Force on Black and Minority Health. Two years later, the task force delivered its report showing that African Americans experienced significantly higher disease rates than whites across six major disease categories—including infant mortality, heart disease, stroke, cancer, and diabetes as well as homicides and accidents. Based on the consistently high rates of disease among African Americans and other minority groups, the DHHS launched the Office of Minority Health in 1987 to provide leadership training and program support to health care agencies and communities to address deep-seated racial disparities in health care.[20]

In 1990, in an important essay on health reforms and the Black community, health researchers R. D. Hester and J. B. Barber called attention to the persistence of racial discrimination in the nation's health care system, forcefully arguing that "a basic health issue in 1990 is the racism that underlies health policy and practices just as it did in 1895. Racism in health in 1990 is perhaps a bit more subtle and less direct than it was in 1895, but possibly even more frustrating because we have a much greater capacity to correct some of the problems" than before. Evidence of blatant racial discrimination resurfaced during the 1980s and 1990s. The color line found sharp expression in the provisions of the Health Care Quality Improvement Act of 1986 (H.R. 5540). This legislation granted "legal immunity to inquisitor physicians against discrimination, defamation of character, or restraint of trade lawsuits, as they carry out the health establishment's peer review and QA policies." As W. Michael Byrd and Linda Clayton make clear, "In American medicine, much of this activity has a sordid history of being racially, socially, and politically motivated (e.g., blocking Black doctors from hospital staff appointments and unfairly disciplining them, eliminating competition among doctors, purging 'unpopular' or 'controversial' doctors from the profession, and enforcing medical establishment agendas)."[21]

Meanwhile, African American physicians, medical students, and patients reported rising levels of overt racial discrimination in the nation's health care system and medical school training programs. In her riveting study of racism in the US medical system, journalist Linda Villarosa recounts the painful story of her own family's encounter with systemic inequality in its quest for equal access to professional health care. In her own words, she recalled her father's hospitalization and treatment at the hands of hospital personnel at Denver's Veterans Administration. When she arrived in town from New York City, where she worked as a reporter for the *New York Times*, she was shocked by what she found: "My father — courtly, sophisticated, and always impeccably dressed — was frighteningly thin, disheveled, wearing a dirty hospital gown, his hair uncombed. Worse, he had restraints on his legs." As she and her father's ex-wife walked into the room, "an attendant was speaking to him in a disrespectful hiss. When I pushed past the attendant and leaned down to hug my father, he whispered, 'Please get me out of here.'"[22]

For Villarosa, her father suffered from a callous racial bias among caregivers of Black patients, particularly those presumed poor and uneducated. When she arrived at the veteran's hospital, her mother bluntly reported, "They are treating your father like a n____; we need to let them see who he is." The two women played the "class card" as a final desperate effort to secure better treatment for their loved one. "We showed them my father's college degree, medals from his military service, and photographs of him pre-illness." In concluding this painful story of Black health care during the postindustrial age, Villarosa explained, "class was the only card my mother and I had so we played it. But like anyone, he should've been treated with dignity."[23]

During the 1990s, the National Medical Association conducted surveys showing that "over 95 percent of African American physicians experienced racial discrimination in their practices on a daily basis," while other studies reported a negative racial environment for some 97 percent of Black students in predominantly white medical schools. As the new century dawned, Byrd and Clayton concluded that "race and class issues in the United States health system still remain to be rectified." By the turn of the twenty-first century, increasing numbers of Black physicians reported closing their practices because of insufficient reimbursements for their services under such federal health programs as Medicare, Medicaid, and third-party payers. In 1990 alone, a study of Black physician practices in North Carolina reported that "between 30 and 40 percent had lost practices." When they closed their doors to patients, many practitioners took paid employment "in emergency rooms in other locations or for health maintenance organizations at significant reductions in income."[24]

Racial integration of the US health care system increased African American access to mainstream medical treatment as well as admission to previously all-white medical schools, but it also resulted in the closing of community-based Black hospitals and clinics that had emerged during the Jim Crow era. These institutions had served, albeit inadequately, the immense health care needs of large numbers of working-class Blacks and provided employment to Black medical professionals. As late as 1982, Black medical schools continued to educate an estimated 25 percent of all Black students seeking professional training in the medical field. But the handwriting on the wall had already signaled the increasing demise of separate Black medical institutions, some schools, and even more hospitals.[25]

In 1979, to take one prominent example, the city of St. Louis closed the famous African American Homer G. Phillips Hospital (HGP). HGP had not only provided essential services to Blacks suffering from various diseases but also trained large numbers of Black medical professionals who in turn helped to broaden African American access to community-based health services. The closing of HGP represented only the tip of a huge iceberg that toppled the industrial-era African American medical infrastructure while failing to incorporate African Americans fully and equally into the expanding postindustrial health care system. At the turn of the new millennium, in their extraordinary two-volume history of African American health care, medical historians Michael Byrd and Linda Clayton conclude that "it is questionable whether" HGP's "production of excellently trained African American" medical professionals "has ever been replaced since its closure in 1979. Certainly, the output of these valuable health professionals in St. Louis and surrounding areas has slowed to a trickle."[26]

By 1990, out of over 400 Black hospitals that had existed over the twentieth century "at one time or another," only eight remained standing at century's end. African American physicians and medical professionals found themselves increasingly pushed to the side as large predominantly white corporate-type medical institutions claimed the capacity to provide "efficient health delivery" services to Black people from "outside the community."[27]

At the same time that the nation closed Black hospitals and medical schools in rising numbers, Black people faced growing restrictions on their access to integrated professional medical school training and the range of medical services to meet the mounting needs of poor and working-class Black patients. Black enrollment in medical schools peaked at 7.5 percent for one year only in 1975. Enrollments declined thereafter, dropping from 43 percent in 1975 to 40 percent in 1980, while the acceptance rate of nonminority students increased from 35 percent in 1974 to 50 percent in 1983. Nationwide, the number of Blacks enrolled in medical schools stagnated between 1978 and 2014, with fewer African American men enrolling in the latter year than the former. This stagnant trend reflected the deleterious impact of conservative reactions against the gains of the Modern Black Freedom Movement.[28]

Conservatives won a major victory in the US Supreme Court's decision in the case of *Regents of the University of California-Davis v. Bakke* (1978). The court ruled that the UC-Davis "special admissions program," which was designed to help close the racial gap in African American and other minorities' access to medical school training, was unconstitutional restriction on the rights of white students seeking admission to the medical school and ordered the admission of Alan Bakke, who had argued that the school's affirmative action program discriminated against him as a white citizen and prospective student. While the court left the door open for universities to use "race" as one consideration in admissions procedures, which encouraged some universities to retain a vigorous recruitment effort focused on increasing minority enrollment, the net effect of the Bakke ruling was to stall progress toward creating a broader and more racially diverse medical profession. African American enrollment not only stagnated across the board but nearly disappeared from the nation's "middle- and lower-ranked schools."[29]

The inadequate integration of African Americans into the nation's medical system, along with the collapse of inner-city Black medical institutions, underscored the precarious foundation of African American life across the class divide in the years after the heyday of the Modern Black Freedom Struggle. Black medical professionals lost access to a relatively protected but segregated and predominantly poor and working-class Black clientele without receiving comparable access to heretofore all-white medical institutions. They also shared with the larger Black middle class a precarious place in the rapidly changing Black urban community. While poor and working-class Blacks bore the lion's share of suffering under the new social welfare order, middle-class and working-class Blacks shared the pain of old and new health challenges within the emerging postindustrial Black urban community. Some studies of Black health and medical care concluded that "the most affluent African Americans in the United States are sicker than the poorest whites." In 2000, a Chicago area study identified and explained the convergence in health care among poor and middle-class Blacks as a product of racially divided housing markets that placed middle-class Blacks in close proximity to the poverty that plagued poor and working-class Black neighborhoods.[30] Such evidence suggests that the cumulative effects of racism and trauma on the physical and psychic well-being of African Americans cut across class lines.

Challenge of New Diseases and Medical Disasters

In varying degrees of intensity, sickle cell anemia, cancer, HIV-AIDS, COVID-19, and Hurricane Katrina posed major challenges to African Americans and the Black medical profession and its white allies. Each major disease followed its own somewhat unique historical trajectory. But they were linked together as significant diseases that invariably took a greater toll on the lives and health of Blacks than whites. They were also tied together by a persistent thread of racial discrimination, insensitivity, and lag in the treatment of African Americans by the mainstream medical profession. Sickle cell anemia, for example, had deep roots in early to mid-twentieth-century African American medical history, but it only gained prominence in the professional medical field during the late twentieth century because of the Modern Black Freedom Movement, among other political, scientific, and medical developments.[31]

Sickle Cell Anemia and Cancer

Medical historian Keith Wailoo forcefully argues that sickle cell anemia received increasing recognition as a scientifically proven and tested genetically inherited disease that reconnected Black people to their origins in west and central Africa. Emerging from the laboratory of the rising field of molecular biology, knowledge of sickle cell anemia also gained stature among scientists and soon attracted attention and money from the federal government. Sickle cell's rising prominence in the scientific and medical world also owed a great deal to innovative breakthroughs in the "use of new antibiotics to treat acute infectious disease."[32]

Still, as Wailoo convincingly concludes, it was "the nationwide struggle over racial segregation and civil rights [that] drove its social visibility, as did the expansion of federally funded biomedical research." At the same time, the movement to eradicate sickle cell anemia became racialized in ways that undercut the rights of the very people it was supposed to help. Medical and government authorities insisted on mandatory testing and related public policies that excluded people with sickle cell anemia from such occupations as flying airplanes, for instance.[33] During the early 1970s, the US Air Force banned people with sickle cell trait from flying, "based on studies suggesting that these otherwise 'normal' people might possibly fall into 'crisis' caused by sickling blood cells when they were deprived of oxygen at high altitude." The military retained this policy until 1984, but die-hard supporters of the ban vigorously campaigned against the policy change, arguing that it violated the military's mission to maintain "an aggressive, efficient, and effecting defense" of the nation.[34]

Cancer offers another prominent case study of race, disease, and challenges to Black health care during the final quarter of the twentieth century. Until the mid-twentieth century, cancer gained attention almost exclusively as a white woman's disease. Only in 1956 did the American Cancer Society acknowledge and make public "the need to take cancer awareness across the color line." The organization finally hired an African American man to "broaden the base of the cancer control movement . . . by working directly with Negro groups and leaders."[35] In early 1970, a team of Howard University researchers discovered a stunning two-decade-long increase in African American deaths from cancer, but this phenomenon had gone undetected by the massive American Cancer Society war on cancer, stretching back to the years before World War I.

Nonetheless, widespread public awareness of cancer as a Black disease only took off after the soul singer Minnie Riperton went public with her battle with cancer in 1977 and finally died two years later. According to *Ebony* magazine, Riperton's battle with cancer transformed her from a model of individual courage and determination to survive into a powerful nationwide symbol of cancer's "growing and tragic destruction of Black people." She became "a metaphor for the tens of thousands of cancer deaths in Black America each year."[36]

HIV-AIDS

The HIV-AIDS epidemic broke out in the early 1980s, but African American AIDS victims were initially marginalized in popular and professional medical discourse on the subject. In 1981, the Centers for Disease Control (CDC) reported the first five cases of HIV-AIDS in the United States, and they were all gay white men. The CDC downplayed evidence that the next four cases were African American men. Early on in the AIDS epidemic, the CDC employed the racialized term "Haitians" to define one high risk segment of the AIDS infected population. This racially biased category remained in force for two years before it was finally abandoned in 1985. At the same time, substantial amounts of sociological and medical research embraced the claim that AIDS "originated in Africa." Researchers and officials in Haiti and Africa challenged these racialized portraits of the disease. As historian David McBride explains, the notion that an African influence underlay "the origins and spread of AIDS" was consistent with a common belief among United States and Western medical researchers that racialized biogenetic factors explained black-white disease differences.[37]

During the late 1980s and early 1990s, the medical establishment gradually acknowledged the growing and alarming racial disparities in HIV-AIDS cases and deaths. By the turn of the new millennium, according to the CDC, African Americans had increased to nearly 50 percent of all AIDS cases in the United States. In the meantime, wealthier and more politically connected white victims of AIDS mobilized their forces, placed pressure on philanthropic and government institutions, and received increasing support for medical help, including new drugs and programs designed to protect the civil rights of gay white men. As these men gained increasing access to necessary resources, they showed little inclination to support their fellow Black gay compatriots. In Philadelphia, however, historian Kevin Mumford shows how Black and White Men Together (BWMT) networks "remained active on a number of fronts of anti-racism."[38]

Hurricane Katrina

In September 2005, a destructive Category 5 hurricane hit the Gulf Coast region of the United States. Hurricane Katrina dramatically exposed the nation's class and racially divided political economy and the very precarious place that African Americans occupied in living environments and the health care system across the country. Katrina and the subsequent flooding of New Orleans when the levees broke claimed the lives of over 1,800 people and forced over a million residents to leave their homes. These residents were disproportionately poor and working-class African Americans living in the city's impoverished Ninth Ward. Decades before the onset of Katrina, poor and working-class whites had largely abandoned the flood-prone Lower

Ninth Ward. They resettled in outlying suburbs, leaving behind an African American population with few alternatives for improving their living space and guarding against catastrophe should the levees break.[39]

In the wake of Hurricane Katrina's destruction, Arnold Hirsch, a prominent urban historian living in New Orleans during the flood, wrote a riveting essay for the *Journal of Urban History* reflecting on his observations and experiences during the storm. He forcefully argued that the tragedy was part of a long history of racial and class inequality in the city of New Orleans, stretching back to the city's origins as a bastion of human bondage during the colonial era. As Hirsch summarized this long history, whites occupied the city's "high ground" while slaves, free Blacks, and immigrants occupied "the lowest, wettest land in a low, wet city." Before the onset of Hurricane Katrina, African Americans made up about 40 percent of the population. Their percentage of the total dropped to about 20 percent in the years following the flood. White resistance to African American movement into previously all-white areas in the region reinforced the mass exodus of Black flood victims from the city. In a 2006 interview on his experience during the flood, social justice activist Malik Rahim described how white flood victims found refuge in the town of Gretna just across the Mississippi River from New Orleans, but Blacks could not: "Once they walked across the bridge, Gretna, and the Jefferson police and the Jefferson Parish police, would turn Blacks around. . . . They would literally tell you, 'Take your Black ass back to the Ninth Ward.'"[40] Moreover, those who managed to reclaim space in the aftermath of the hurricane confronted a profound decline in their access to medical care.[41]

On the eve of Katrina, the Louisiana State University Medical Center managed two hospitals—Charity Hospital and the University Hospital. African Americans comprised 75 percent of patients at Charity, over half without the benefit of health insurance, compared to the extreme opposite at University Hospital, where 96 percent of patients reported health insurance. Following the storm, however, only University Hospital reopened, leaving African American residents in a more precarious health predicament than before. Before the storm, Charity Hospital had not only provided care for HIV-AIDS victims, alcoholism and drug abuse, and trauma; it had also served as a training ground and employer for thousands of city and state resident physicians, nurses, and other health care professionals.[42]

In the winter and spring of 2020, the onset of the coronavirus pandemic opened a new chapter in the history of race, disease, and medicine in American and African American history. Compared to several other countries, the United States delayed its response to the spreading pandemic until many people had perished. Only then did the US government institute measures (social distancing, accent on personal hygiene like handwashing, and curtailment of large social gatherings) to arrest the destructive impact of the virus.[43] During a virtual town hall meeting on the crisis sponsored by the New York Urban League, Jumaane Williams, New York City's Public Advocate, declared that "every step of the way we have been so far behind. . . . We should have shut down the city and been utilizing the Emergency Broadcast System and Zoned the city so we could deliver food to those who needed it." Similarly, Marc Morial, president and CEO of the National Urban League, decried what he called "fake information that the disease would not affect African Americans." He also implored the CDC "in each and every state to gather accurate information on every person who has been infected and those who have unfortunately passed."[44]

COVID-19

Mounting evidence of alarming racial disparities quickly demolished the foundation of erroneous early reports. Research on the racial impact of COVID-19 soon dispelled the notion that Blacks were less susceptible to the disease; in fact, the research demonstrated that Black people were disproportionately represented among those contracting the disease and dying from the pandemic. By early April, Louisiana's Black population accounted for 70 percent of COVID deaths, although Blacks made up only 32 percent of the state's total population. Similarly, with only 13 percent of the state's population, Michigan's Black communities reported 40 percent of the deaths. For its part, Chicago reported African Americans "dying from coronavirus at six times the rate of whites." As late as July 2023, in North Carolina, African Americans made up 22 percent of the state's total population, but they accounted for 36 percent of the state's COVID deaths, while Latinos, making up just under 10 percent of the total population, accounted for 17 percent of the deaths. Together, North Carolina's African American and Latinx population registered 87 percent of food production workers, 67 percent of food service workers, 58 percent of construction workers, and 44 percent of all health care workers who perished during the pandemic. Black people not only died in disproportionately higher numbers than whites, they also died at younger ages.[45]

Popular media and academic discussions soon started to acknowledge how the historic concentration of African Americans in dangerous and unhealthy work and living environments, as well the persistence of racial inequality in medical science and health care practices, exposed them to disproportionately higher disease and death rates than their Euro-American counterparts. Racially segregated housing markets, for example, curtailed African American access to nutritious foods and healthy green spaces. Environmental activists regularly describe poor and working-class Black neighborhoods as "food deserts" without adequate access to grocery stores with fresh fruits and vegetables. Conversely, other scholars note that poor and working-class communities were also often sites of "food swamps" with an excessive number of fast-food outlets like McDonald's and Burger King. Environmental obstacles to fresh food exacerbated and reinforced a litany of preexisting conditions (diabetes, heart disease, and kidney failure, to name few) that fueled "the higher rates of African Americans contracting the coronavirus."[46]

Work and workplaces also put African Americans at higher risk of contracting the coronavirus than their white brothers and sisters. Large numbers of African Americans work in service-sector jobs that cannot be performed at home in quarantine to protect themselves and their families from the disease. Cecilia Munoz, a domestic policy adviser in President Barack Obama's administration, noted that these workers cannot stare at computer screens all day long. They must go out there into the workplace and give it their all as "janitors, caregivers, grocery store workers, first responders and of course hospital workers." Nationwide, 20 percent of Black workers and 16 percent of Latino workers occupied jobs where they could work remotely compared to 30 percent of white workers. Black and Latino workers must also drive the buses, trucks, and trains that transport people and necessary supplies to their destinations. As Munoz powerfully concludes, the coronavirus has upended our conventional notions about who are "essential workers." Specifically, it has brought these ordinarily "invisible" workers into "plain sight" as the linchpin of our survival as a people during this worldwide crisis.[47]

Even as Black and white workers gradually received public recognition as "essential workers" during the era of the coronavirus, their jobs were by no means secure. As the pandemic took hold and public health officials closed schools, restaurants, and other public places, employers laid off rising numbers of workers. African Americans were disproportionately represented among the unemployed. In February, for a brief moment, when the United States declared the pandemic a national public health emergency and ordered businesses and public places to close, the long-standing Black unemployment number that was double that of white workers declined slightly, but it soon returned to the "traditional two-to-one ratio." Between February and April 2020, some 40 percent of Black-owned businesses also closed their doors. On the eve of the pandemic, the Federal Reserve Bank of New York had reported 58 percent of Black-owned enterprises at risk of closing compared to 27 percent for white businesses.[48]

Meanwhile, Black people who contracted the disease soon reported discriminatory treatment in hospitals and clinics charged with treating COVID-19 patients. Some recent studies show that African American patients "receive poorer quality health care" than whites in the nation's hospitals, clinics, and federally funded rescue projects. In a painful video that went viral in December 2020, a Black physician, Dr. Susan Moore, claimed "implicit" racial bias by a white physician at an Indiana hospital. Shortly after relocating to another facility, Moore died apparently from "COVID-19 complications." Melanie Campbell, president of the National Coalition on Black Civic Participation and a COVID-19 survivor, implored the federal COVID-19 task force to "pay special attention to what is happening with racial disparities in hospital care, especially as it relates to who is admitted when they show up for treatment based on race and gender."[49]

When public health officials approved the rollout of the Moderna and Pfizer COVID-19 vaccines, the process quickly became racialized. Although roughly the same percentage of Blacks (39 percent) and whites (36 percent) reported that they wanted to delay taking the shot, health authorities focused attention on "educating black people about the vaccine," while moving ahead and actually "vaccinating white people." In their important study of racial health disparities during the pandemic, health researchers Keisha L. Bentley-Edwards, Melissa J. Scott, and Paul A. Robbins concluded that the COVID-19 pandemic, especially the vaccine rollout, "crystallized the need for racial equity in health implementation strategies and health communications."[50]

In March 2020, when the federal government passed the Coronavirus Aid, Relief, and Economic Security (CARES) Act, the largest relief package (at $2.2 trillion) in the nation's history, relief unfolded along the unequal color line. According to a Brookings Institute study, African Americans were disproportionately represented among those who received delayed rather than prompt payment. These groups — renters, people without bank accounts, and people with low income and low assets — all faced difficulties gaining payment under the CARES legislation. CARES administrator placed priority on paying people "whose bank information (from recent tax filings) had been stored with the Internal Revenue Service." A similar process characterized the federal Paycheck Protection Program (PPP). This program provided low interest loans to businesses in order "to continue paying their employees and meet other business costs." However, as Lucas Hubbard, Gwendolyn Wright, William Darity, and other scholars of race and the pandemic noted, "rather than help the poor," PPP funds "delivered most of its benefits to the already wealthy" and predominantly white businesspeople and their employees.[51]

Mental Health and the Carceral State

By the late twentieth and early twenty-first century, the psychiatry profession reported an alarming drop in available beds for mental health patients. The number of beds had dropped from 337 per 100,000 population in 1955 to only about 30 beds per 100,000 in 2014.[52] The vast majority of beds devoted to psychiatric treatment in the United States had migrated to prisons, jails, and homeless shelters. Chicago's Cook County Jail accounts for the country's largest number of patients (predominantly Black) receiving on-site psychiatric treatment. At the historic and infamous Milledgeville State Hospital in Georgia, authorities converted ten buildings into "five maximum-security prisons, giving Georgia in the early 1990s the second largest such conversion rate in the United States." At a statewide meeting of mental health professionals in Georgia, Baldwin County commissioner Henry Craig lamented the increasing dearth of treatment for the mentally ill outside the prison walls. As he put it, "We have a moral issue. . . . When a person is mentally ill, too often, [that person] goes to jail and the criminal justice system provides the help that the community, the families, the government did not provide. Our judicial law enforcement know that it's morally wrong. . . . We need to find a different solution for those that are ill with mental illness—keyword, ill."[53]

During the late 1960s and early 1970s, new equal rights legislation increased medical services for mental health patients, but the digital age regime soon severely undercut resources for the mentally ill. In 2017, the American Psychiatric Association noted that reported cases of mental disorders are "similar" or even "fewer" among African Americans than among whites, but African American cases may persist over a longer period of time. However, other recent studies of mental illness are giving greater attention to the dearth of knowledge on the issue of "stress" among African Americans, particularly given the highly discriminatory, violent, and hazardous conditions under which African Americans, particularly poor and working-class Black youth and adults, live and work.[54]

In the wake of the African American health crisis in the expanding postindustrial city, African Americans turned again to their community-based networks and forged creative new responses to ongoing but shifting health challenges. Digital age Black activism not only included the medical work of established churches and civil rights, political, and social service organizations. It also included the activities of essential workers at the bottom of the new economy's workforce.

Long Medical Rights Movement

Black service workers were by no means quiescent in the throes of the deindustrializing economy and the increasing erosion of worker rights and benefits. Between 1969 and 1989, an interracial group of Black and white health care workers built a substantial union—Local "1199." It had deep roots and abiding ties to the parent body, the New York City Local 1199, founded under the leadership of a Russian immigrant named Leon Davis. From the outset of its formation during the turbulent years of the Great Depression through the late twentieth century, 1199 articulated an abiding belief in organizing the most "marginalized workers in the hospital industry—Blacks, Puerto Ricans, poor whites, [and] women."[55]

Poor and Working-Class Blacks Organize

Grassroots organizing gained powerful expression when the New York City–based Local 1199 took the advice of Coretta Scott King and other civil rights leaders and moved their organizing efforts beyond New York City to other Northern and Southern cities as well as the southern Appalachian coalfields. Under the banner of 1199, African Americans joined forces with white health care workers and launched strike actions against the Presbyterian University Hospital in Pittsburgh, the Clinch Valley Clinic Hospital in Richlands, Virginia, and most notably the Medical College Hospital of Charleston, South Carolina. The organization focused its attention on improving the lives of "orderlies; and dietary, maintenance, housekeeping, and laundry workers."[56]

While Black and white hospital workers gained few tangible benefits from their struggles against giant hospital systems in their cities and regions, they nonetheless demonstrated the capacity of interracial groups of workers to wage collective actions on their own behalf. In Charleston, South Carolina, the union conducted a four-month-long strike in the face of stiff company

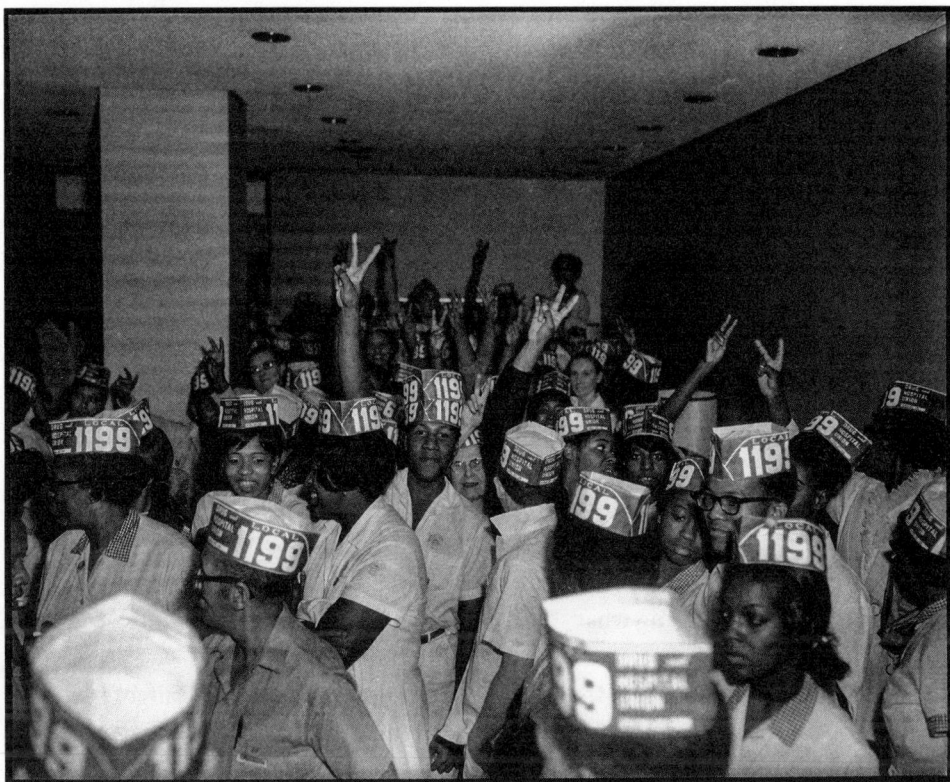

Pittsburgh workers wearing "Local 1199" hats and displaying the V for Victory sign, celebrating the union's hard-fought battle for recognition at the city's Presbyterian University Hospital. Charles "Teenie" Harris/Carnegie Museum of Art, via Getty Images.

resistance, backed up by state and local police power, including the arrest of several movement activists. Although the union failed to negotiate a formal contract, it did gain a "memorandum of agreement." Medical College Hospital reinstated fired union members, increased the wages of workers, established a grievance procedure, and promised to set up a credit union to serve the needs of hospital workers. Coretta Scott King played a major role in the Charleston strike and supported unionizing efforts elsewhere through personal appearances and speeches under the organizing motto "Union Power, Soul Power," linking the civil rights, labor, and medical rights movements.[57]

Under the leadership of Aid to Families with Dependent Children (AFDC) recipient Margaret "Peggy" McCarty, the first chair of an activist group called Mother Rescuers, residents of Baltimore's Black public housing staged a rent strike to protest and demand rectification of the dilapidated and rat-infested

O'Donnell Heights Housing project. Although the rent strike stopped short of majority support from residents, it underscored the ongoing struggle of poor and working-class women to change the conditions under which they and their families lived. The protesters enlisted the help of legal aid lawyers, exposed the hazardous conditions at the complex, and set the groundwork for the city's receipt of a $30.1 million federal grant in 1981 to improve its dilapidated public housing stock.[58]

In 1983, under the leadership of Roxanne Jones, poor and working-class Black Philadelphians staged a sit-in at the Philadelphia Gas Works to protest the increasing termination of service to poor families unable to pay their fuel bills. And in Watts, Brooklyn, and Philadelphia, grassroots activist women fueled the development of government and foundation-funded Community Development Corporations. For a brief moment, these organizations creatively addressed the challenges of unhealthy and unsafe living conditions in Black neighborhoods — not by flight but by rebuilding. As such, they advanced an agenda that historian Brian Purnell describes as the "unmaking" of the ghetto, including what some analysts called the "medical ghetto."[59]

Following the shooting death of her sixteen-year-old son in Detroit in 1986, Clementine Barfield founded SOSAD (Save Our Sons and Daughters) "to go beyond mourning" and "create positive alternatives to violence throughout the community." In Los Angeles, Black women formed Mothers ROC (Reclaiming Our Children) and Mothers of East Los Angeles (MELA). These organizations not only aimed to curb Black on Black violence but also worked to find jobs for young men and to help those caught in the throes of the racially biased criminal justice system. When the state of California proposed to build a prison in East Los Angeles, MELA, founded in 1984, joined forces with the Latino community and blocked the project. MELA also thwarted plans to build a hazardous waste incinerator in the area.[60]

Medical Justice Activists, Social Welfare Professionals, and Public Officials

In significant ways, as the African American health crisis intensified during the 1980s and 1990s, Black medical justice leaders turned inward and pushed for the resources to expand and even increase the number of medical schools and community-based hospitals serving the African American community. Dr. Louis W. Sullivan, the second African American secretary of the US Department of Housing and Human Services, spearheaded the development of the much-needed Morehouse School of Medicine and led the effort to establish permanent branches of the National Institutes of Health (NIH) and the National Cancer Institute (NCI) to address minority health issues. Similarly, Dr. David Satcher, the first African American selected to head the CDC, played a pivotal role in preventing the closure of historic Meharry Medical College, the nation's "oldest, largest, African American medical school," during his tenure as president during the 1980s.[61]

Likewise, Dr. Joycelyn Elders, a pediatrician and first African American US Surgeon General, appointed during the Clinton administration, emerged as a major advocate for the resuscitation of historic community-based Black medical institutions as a way out of the contemporary Black health crisis. In an important essay on diabetes in the Black community, Elders and her coauthor Frederick Murray forcefully argued for the redevelopment of a strong Black community-based medical infrastructure, with abiding ties to African American religious, political, entrepreneurial, educational, and social service organizations.[62]

Local branches of the National Urban League played a major role in helping poor and working-class Blacks navigate the socioeconomic and health challenges of the postindustrial city. The Urban League of Pittsburgh (ULP), for example, created a variety of programs for improving the housing, health, and diets for thousands of poor and working-class Blacks and their families.[63] In 2009–10, the ULP opened a new Health Education Office (HEO) and announced a new health initiative called "Newer Thrusts in Health Care." The HEO underscored continuing racial disparities in the city's health care system, including "critical shortages of physicians, dentists and other specialized" health care providers; "continued defects" in the utilization of prevailing medical facilities and services; and the rising costs of medical care in general. Formed through a collaboration with the University of Pittsburgh's School of Nursing and its Clinical and Translational Science Institute, the center served over 600 clients in its first year. Under the leadership of staff member Kafui Agbemenu, a registered nurse and PhD student in nursing at the University of Pittsburgh, the HEO offered basic health screenings for blood pressure, weight, and cancer. The center also provided preventive care services, including flu shots, nutrition classes, and CPR training.[64]

To strengthen and reinforce its health care programs, the ULP also developed food support projects to help poor and working-class Black families. The hunger services staff and the health advocate developed a nutrition program for young people to improve their "understanding of nutrition and of food selection and preparation." This program offered the expert advice of Judy Dodd, dietitian in the Nutrition Science Department at the University of Pittsburgh; classes in nutrition taught by a graduate student in the nutrition and sciences field; and a demonstration of food art by students from the Pennsylvania Culinary Institute. By 2010–11, the Hunger Services Pantry, located at the Wood Street Office of the ULP, provided emergency food supplies to nearly 800 families. In the meantime, the league's annual Thanksgiving Food distribution program had emerged as "one of the most successful food programs in the region."[65]

Medical justice activists also opened new fronts of protests against hazardous living conditions, environmental injustice, and what they defined as "environmental racism." In 1987, the United Church of Christ Commission for Racial Justice published its study *Toxic Wastes and Race in the United States*. This study documented the siting of toxic waste dumps in Black neighborhoods and helped to spearhead the emergence of the environmental justice movement and its commitment to eradicate "environmental racism." These efforts included spirited movements to combat lead poisoning, secure assistance for single women with children, create programs to end youth violence and rising levels of Black on Black homicides, and urge public officials to enact new legislation and social policies designed to end police brutality and the murder of Black citizens in police custody.[66]

Cross-class poor, working-class, and professional organizing campaigns inspired the emergence of a new and more energetic Black urban medical rights politics by century's end. In city after city, African Americans built multiracial coalitions with liberal whites as well as Latino/Latina Americans and Asian American voters. They articulated a clear vision for building a fairer urban social order than existed under the leadership of predominantly white Democratic and Republican political machines. By the opening of the new millennium, African Americans had won the mayor's office in such diverse cities as Detroit, New Orleans, Philadelphia, Atlanta, Los Angeles, New York, and Chicago.[67] In the wake of the expanding health crisis, African Americans and their multiracial and ethnic allies pushed for passage of national health insurance as the surest way to support improvements in health and health care among Blacks and the nation's poor and working classes. As such, they supported Jesse Jackson's campaigns to become the Democratic Party's nominee for president. Integral to Jackson's quest for his party's nomination was a plan for universal health insurance. His plan would replace private health insurance plans with a single government-funded plan. Following Jackson's defeat for the Democratic Party's nomination in 1984 and again in 1988, a variety of market-oriented health insurance programs—most notably, health maintenance organizations (HMOs)—took center stage in the quest to reform the nation's health system. HMOs embodied a system of "for profit" health care organizations fueled by large infusions of federal dollars that undermined the quality of health care available to African Americans as well as the medical practices of Black doctors.[68]

Expanding the Scope and Diversifying Responses to the Health Care Crisis

Closely intertwined with a variety of multifaceted social justice campaigns, postindustrial Black medical professionals and their intraracial and interracial allies also spearheaded a series of medical rights movements focused on the intersecting and overlapping struggles against sickle cell anemia, cancer, AIDS, and the coronavirus, among many other aspects of the African American health crisis. But these struggles were by no means uniform across all categories of medical inequality. Despite the extraordinary outpouring of support for sickle cell research and the quest for a cure, for example, some medical care activists and political leaders questioned the high priority placed on federal dollars for the project. They worried that the professional self-interest of the white medical establishment motivated the push for sickle cell funding without regard to the overall health needs of the Black community. Members of the Congressional Black Caucus (CBC) voiced their concerns. In April 1972, the CBC supported passage of the National Sickle Cell Anemia Control Act, but it roundly condemned what it described as "the twisted priorities of government and grant-making institutes." According to the CBC, sickle cell anemia did not deserve top billing in the fight for better health for Black people, "when essentially hypertension kills more Blacks in one year than Sickle Cell in twenty."[69] Still, the Black medical rights movement helped to fuel the federal government and the medical profession's growing support for the fight against sickle cell anemia.

Unlike the fight against sickle cell anemia, the struggle against cancer gained widespread popular support within the African American community but only gradually attracted the attention of the mainstream medical, scientific, and philanthropic community. Following the pioneering Howard University study of cancer mortality rates among Black people, the fight against cancer soon gradually emerged as a major priority in the medical rights movement. In the wake of the Howard report, research on various facets of race and cancer continued to unfold, all offering additional support for the argument that African Americans not only shouldered an "unequal burden of cancer" but also endured "unequal treatment."[70]

Symbolizing the growing influence of the African American medical rights movement, Dr. La Salle Leffal, a surgeon and chief architect of the Howard cancer study, became the first African American president of the American Cancer Society in 1978. Much like other medical and social struggles of the postindustrial era, the fight against cancer had antecedents in the early twentieth-century campaigns against medical apartheid. Keith Wailoo succinctly notes that the "roots of this new awareness of a democratic cancer in the 1970s—in epidemiology, in cultural representation, and in awareness— had been laid by the social changes of the 1960s and by economic and cultural shifts many decades earlier."[71]

If some African Americans provided lukewarm support for massive federal programs to fight sickle cell anemia and others enthusiastically embraced the fight against cancer, large sectors of the Black community remained silent at the outset of the HIV-AIDS crisis. Unlike the vigorous community-based African American campaigns to stop the spread of tuberculosis (TB), the late twentieth-century Black community was exceedingly slow to mobilize grassroots support to address the AIDS health crisis. As late as 1988, in New York City, the commissioner of health surveyed the range of community resources available to fight the AIDS epidemic. Among the community-based programs identified as AIDS victims advocacy or support groups, not one was "specifically operated by predominantly black organizations" or even the city's Black AIDS community itself.[72]

Some Black ministers and their congregations were not merely silent, but they actively opposed efforts to alleviate the suffering of AIDS victims. In Boston's Black Roxbury community, Reverend Graylon Ellis-Hagler mobilized opposition to a local needle-exchange program. When Ellis-Hagler and members of his congregation "picketed the site," police moved in and closed the project. The CBC also remained largely silent on the AIDS crisis until the early 1990s, when outstanding pro-basketball legend Earvin "Magic" Johnson publicly announced that he had tested HIV-positive. These members of Congress soon became avid fighter for federal resources to support the quest for a cure and services for Black AIDS victims, including protests over the CDC's plan to slash some $14 million from the budget of AIDS advocacy groups working among African American and other minority communities.[73]

Gradually, the African American community embraced the fight against AIDS and established a growing range of programs to combat the disease across the country. Beginning slowly during the late 1980s and early 1990s, the African American community initiated an expanding number of HIV-AIDS assistance programs by working with ministers of New York City's largest African American churches and San Francisco's Black Coalition on AIDS, among other groups across the country. But it was the Black AIDS community itself that led the way. In the wake of the HIV-AIDS epidemic, gay Black men gradually organized their own grassroots movement to call attention to their plight. They fought an uphill battle not only against the grain of the white gay rights movement but also against the grain of anti-gay sentiment within the Black community itself.[74]

As in other epidemics, gay Black men had to mobilize themselves and enlist the African American community in their struggle for equal access to services available to treat and cure the AIDS virus. By the early twentieth century, they had formed such organizations as the National Black Leadership Commission on AIDS (NBLCA), Balm in Gilead, the Black AIDS Institute, and the New York–based Gay Men of African Descent (GMAD), to name a few. Only as the Black gay community organized its own movement, supplemented by the gradual involvement of the larger African American community, would African Americans gradually enter the network of medical and social services for victims of HIV-AIDS.[75]

In the aftermath of Hurricane Katrina, the city's Black population in New Orleans persevered, despite massive displacement to various locales across the country. They tapped into a rich history of wisdom, knowledge, and strength reaching back to the city's founding. Within days of the peak floodwaters, activists in the Algiers neighborhood formed the Common Ground health clinic. The clinic reported that some 4,000 people visited the clinic during the first two months of its operation. According to founder member of the organization, Malik Rahim, "Right after the hurricane, we came to the realization that the city wasn't going to provide any services. . . . So under that environment of blatant racism and total abandonment by the federal government, we founded Common Ground."[76]

But the struggle to reclaim and maintain homes in New Orleans was a perennial uphill climb. Nonetheless, as suggested by the launch of Common Ground, victims of Hurricane Katrina were no less active than their forebears in their own effort to return to their homes, rebuild, and reclaim space in the Crescent City. From the outset of the calamity, poor and working-class Black residents forged their own widely held interpretation of the disaster. They refused to believe that levees broke on their own volition. They sought the hand of man in the destruction that they faced. In an exceedingly revealing essay on grassroots African American interpretation of their lives in the wake of Katrina, historian Ari Kelman notes how the city's Black working class drew upon their historical memory of an earlier moment when powerful elites manufactured the bombing of the levees to save their own homes from floodwaters.[77]

Kelman examines the origins of the "rumor" that the government dynamited the levees that flooded the Ninth Ward in order to protect white neighborhoods from devastation by the storm. Kelman convincingly argues that the rumor emerged from the grassroots of the Ninth Ward's Black community and that certain historical events gave the rumors credence and fomented widespread belief rather than disbelief within Black New Orleans. From the outset of the city's history as a slave-trading center of the French empire, the New Orleans levees (constructed and maintained in part by slave and convict labor) symbolized the intertwining of race and class inequality in the lives of Black residents. During the late nineteenth and twentieth centuries, technological innovations and new federal programs enabled the construction of higher levees, better pumps, and elaborate drainage systems. Kelman documents how technological changes and massive government investments in flood control projects presumably made the levees more trustworthy, but again and again predominantly poor and working-class Black neighborhoods suffered disproportionate inundation when the pumps or levees failed.[78]

In 1927, an elite-dominated organization called the ad hoc Citizen Flood Relief Committee (CFRC) defied the law and blew up the levee some twenty miles downstream of the city of New Orleans. The explosion forced hundreds of poor people to evacuate their homes and abandon their land without later receiving adequate compensation. Victims of the 1927 flood later filed a series of lawsuits that expressed and fueled a widespread belief—that the city's economic and political elites would protect their own interests at any cost, including "manufacturing a flood" to divert stormwaters away from their own neighborhoods and businesses. In the wake of Hurricane Betsy in 1968 and Katrina in 2005, the historical memory of race and class injustice again produced suspicions and charges that city officials had dynamited the levees in order to keep white upper-class communities dry. Thus, Kelman concludes that the levee rumors persisted among Ninth Ward residents because "they knew that the disaster they survived was unnatural, and that as long as people insisted it was, little would change to insure that such a thing would not happen again."[79]

Literary and cultural studies scholar Farah Jasmine Griffin examines the meaning of Katrina as part of a long-term historical process of "human rights violations," on the one hand, and a corresponding process of "human resilience and resistance," on the other. She analyzes these issues through the lens of "culture and music," emphasizing how Black artists, intellectuals, musicians, and performers regularly articulated themes of disaster, abandonment, dislocation, and dispersal in their works. Drawing upon the conceptual insights of psychiatrist Mindy Thompson Fullilove's notion of "root shock" (i.e., the "human trauma" that accompanied the displacement of hundreds of urban Blacks during the era of urban renewal), Griffin illustrates these themes through the novels of Nobel laureate Toni Morrison, the lyrics of early twentieth-century blues woman Bessie Smith, and the autobiography of well-known musician Sidney Bechet.[80]

Griffin urges us to remember the history of African American creativity as a context for understanding post-Katrina New Orleans and encouraging responses of hope for the future of the city. In her view, Black New Orleans was not only the product of African dispersal through the slave trade but also subsequent dispersals associated with the Haitian Revolution, the emergence of maroon communities in the swamps around the city, and the great twentieth-century Black migration into and out of the city. Bursts of creativity accompanied each moment of communal rupture: Congo Square during the French colonial era; the emergence of alternative African American Mardi Gras Indian celebrations during the emancipation era; blues, jazz, rhythm and blues, and hip-hop during the twentieth century. In other words, "African influences shaped the cultures of the Americas while at the same time reflecting the trauma of having been torn from their native home, stripped of kin and community, forced to labor without pay and subjected to unimaginable acts of physical, spiritual and psychic violence."[81]

For her part, Danille Taylor, dean of the humanities at Dillard University in New Orleans, reflects on the political, institutional, and personal meanings of Katrina one year after the tragedy. While the storm destroyed much of her home, it devastated Dillard University, her workplace and primary institutional affiliation. Similar to Hirsch, Kelman, and Griffin, Taylor argues that the legacy of political corruption, social injustice, and economic inequality in New Orleans and the state of Louisiana ensured that the poor and the working class would not only endure the brunt of Katrina's damage but also face an unequal footing for rebuilding their lives in the hurricane's aftermath. In her view, Mayor Ray Nagin had failed to address the city's joblessness, poor housing, inadequate education, and escalating murder rate on the eve of the disaster. Only "after the hurricane," she maintains, did Nagin become a kind of "folk hero" when he declared in his Martin Luther King Day speech of 2006 that the "Chocolate City" would rise again.[82]

Despite the surge in Nagin's popularity, Taylor concludes that his policies in the aftermath of Katrina fell far short of a comprehensive plan to rebuild the city and ensure that the levees would hold against future Katrinas. As she puts it, "The Mayor's 'blue chip' commission generated a planning report that has been ignored and sits on a shelf because of the lack of citizens' response." Thus, alongside other local efforts to bring the city's scattered African American population back home, Taylor firmly believes that the rebuilding of Dillard will represent a key beacon in the return migration of Black New Orleanians from the diaspora back to the Crescent City. In August 2015, a broad cross-section of the New Orleans community met to commemorate the tenth anniversary of Hurricane Katrina and to reflect on their own survival and future in the city. A substantial portion of the festivities focused on "wellness programs, health screenings, and interfaith support," underscoring the determination among Katrina survivors to face the future with hope and faith.[83]

If Hurricane Katrina tested the faith of survivors, the onset of COVID-19 posed even greater challenges to established churches and the faith of Black Americans. In the COVID-19 era, Blacks employed their religious beliefs to aid their responses to the twenty-first-century African American health crisis, as they had done in earlier periods of history. While their beliefs in the efficacy of professional medical care continued to expand, they remained deeply embedded within the fabric of the African American church. In her groundbreaking study of Black Christianity amid the pandemic, sociologist Sandra Barnes explores the lives of a single Black family, the Marshalls (a pseudonym), to ascertain the possible impact of COVID-19 on their religious ideas and practices. While some members of the Marshall family reported that the pandemic had little impact on their prior religious beliefs and practices, most claimed that the pandemic strengthened their religiosity, prayer, and Bible study. Through numerous interviews with members of the Marshall family, Barnes illustrates how the closing of Black churches and transition to online services virtually eliminated a key pillar of the long struggle against persisting patterns of class and racial inequality in the larger political economy of the nation and neighborhoods. As she puts it, "Churches have historically been sanctuaries in the Black community to help negotiate disparities, [and] ordinarily, they would likely have played an important role as blacks navigated the pandemic and protests about police violence. Thus, for some blacks, closed churches may be just as damaging as opened ones."[84]

Furthermore, Barnes calls for much more attention to the ways that "today's churches may help combat health issues, foster activism against social problems," and calm the nerves of followers as they manage their lives amid crisis times. Indeed, she offers the telling illustration of one male family member who clearly articulated a profound sense of loss following the closure of his church and move toward virtual services. In his own words, the fifty-two-year-old administrator with an MBA degree declared, "My mind races now—church used to help calm me down. I'm worried about a lot—my Mom, [who's] recovering from a heart attack, Covid-19, and now George Floyd. He represents all those black people who have been killed—going back to Emmett Till. . . . I've been stopped by cops too many times to remember. I pray for the protesters every day. Sometimes I think, if Rona [coronavirus] doesn't get us, the cops will." Many other Marshall family members expressed their deeply held faith that God would see them through the pandemic. Lola, a fifty-six-year-old marketing analyst declared her belief, succinctly and pointedly, that God provided her with a reliable shield against the virus. "There's going to be hundreds and even ten thousand that fall by my side. I know this sounds bad, but He has me."[85]

As hard as proponents of modern scientific-based medicine may have worked to stamp out traditional communal medical practices among African Americans, over more than a century later, such beliefs and practices held on. Under crisis conditions like HIV-AIDS and the coronavirus, they also witnessed a vigorous revival among poor and working-class Blacks and even some professionals, including nurses, as suggested by the career of nurse Linda Janet Holmes. In her important book *Safe in a Midwife's Hands: Birthing Traditions from Africa to the American South* (2023), Holmes urges a return to the home for childbirth among Black women. In 1981, she moved to Alabama under a research grant from the National Endowment for the Humanities. Over a six-month period, she conducted interviews with African American midwives who had practiced their craft over a lifetime during the Jim Crow era. Across the spectrum of interviews, she identified a set of core beliefs that guided the work of these women. Over and over again, the women urged their patients to remain active during labor, stay awake and aware of the birthing process, and welcome others to the birthing room "to provide comfort throughout the birthing process." During the late twentieth and early twenty-first century, Holmes emerged as an activist in the "birthing justice movement." She aimed to help women recover the ancient knowledge of home and community-based childbirth—to avoid what she describes as the perils of hospital delivery in predominantly white environments that are especially hostile to Black women. Key to unlocking this knowledge and advancing the fight "to end inequities in birthing care and outcomes," she powerfully argues, is a profound belief in God. As she puts it, "Midwives taught me how to talk to God."[86]

With the outbreak of the coronavirus, the Black Lives Matter Movement (BLM) helped to spearhead the development of new organizations designed to address the challenges of the pandemic. Following the national conventions of the Republican and Democratic parties in the summer of 2020, a coalition of over a hundred groups joined the Black Lives Matter Electoral Justice Project. Ahead of the general election, the organization convened the 2020 Black National Convention. Held virtually, the convention attracted close to 500,000 participants. Activists repeatedly underscored the significance of community-based organizing and institutions for the long-term success of movements designed to eradicate systemic inequality and social injustice. Spencer Overton, president of the Joint Center for Political and Economic Studies, reiterated this point in an interview on the subject. "Any battle plan for progress," he said, "must incorporate building and fortifying Black institutions. . . . Strong Black institutions allow us to weather the storms, exercise agency and leadership, debate, participate and fully take advantage of opportunities."[87]

In 2022, the National Center for Health Statistics, a division of the CDC, reported a two-year decline in the nation's overall life expectancy, a product of the destructive impact of COVID-19. But Black life expectancy had declined by 0.7 years compared to a larger drop for Native Americans (two years) and the Euro-American population (a full year). According to Reed Tuckson, cofounder of the Black Coalition Against COVID and a former Washington, DC, commissioner of public health, the lower rate of decline for African Americans reflected the "extraordinary efforts made by the Black community to overcome the excess burden of death" that plagued the African American community at the outset of the pandemic.[88]

In the presidential election of 2020, the creative organizing efforts of the African American community helped to elect Joe Biden, vice president during the Obama era, to the president's office. Republicans had pledged to demolish the comprehensive Patient Protection and Affordable Care Act (ACA) of 2010, popularly known as Obamacare. Now African Americans reclaimed a measure of hope. Biden and his vice president Kamala Harris, an African American woman, not only promised aggressive steps to end the pandemic but also to preserve and even expand the benefits of the ACA to poor and working-class Americans across the color line. As the Biden term ended, the nation and the African American community claimed a few salient victories in the health field, but the results were insufficient to reverse the effects of centuries of medical apartheid, aggravated by the impact of a new worldwide pandemic.[89]

Despite the profound limits of the new politics for adequately meeting the medical and other needs of poor and working-class Black families and their communities, Black mayoral regimes and the subsequent election and reelection of Barack H. Obama as the first US president of African descent benefited from the energy, enthusiasm, and support of poor and working-class Black voters. The passage of the ACA and establishment of a new health insurance program reduced the number of uninsured Americans from nearly 50 million in 2010 to about 30 million by 2016. This included an estimated 3 million Blacks and 4 million Latinx people who were previously uninsured. By extending much-needed medical insurance to poor and working-class families, Obamacare reinforced grassroots support for Obama's reelection in 2012.[90]

After Obama's reelection, increasing deaths of young African Americans in police custody underlay the groundswell of grassroots activism that launched Black Lives Matter in 2013. Following the acquittal of George Zimmerman in the shooting death of unarmed Trayvon Martin in Sanford, Florida, a gated suburban community, BLM not only staged massive street protests but also established some twenty-five organized local chapters across the country. After the 2016 presidential election and the triumph of the most conservative wing of the Republican Party, massive street protests broke out in cities nationwide. But many Black Lives Matter activists also called for deeper and more extensive engagement in the established electoral political process. Alicia Garza, a pioneer in the development of BLM as well as an organizer for the National Domestic Worker's Alliance, reported "doing a lot of work to build bridges between other movements and communities caught in the crosshairs of [Donald] Trump's agenda."[91]

Meanwhile, ahead of the 2020 presidential election, the murder of George Floyd by a Minneapolis police officer not only reinforced the broader fight for social justice for Black people but also underscored escalating police violence against young Black men and women as a public health crisis. As historian Jay D. Aronson and physician Roger A. Mitchell note in their book on the subject, the United States has devised "one of the most advanced vital records systems in the world." Yet, it has failed to produce an accurate accounting of the mounting deaths of African Americans in police custody. In their view, it seems, ignorance of the precise magnitude of this human and civil rights violation "is not accidental" but "intentional, officially sanctioned, and officially produced."[92] Although the death of George Floyd in police custody touched off the largest global protests in the history of the world, the fight for social justice, mental and physical safety, and well-being continues as we wrap up the first quarter of the twenty-first century.

Conclusion

As the new millennium entered its third decade, poor and working-class African Americans occupied the bottom ranks of the nation's expanding high-tech service economy. As they left manufacturing jobs behind, they received low wages and few benefits in the form of health insurance and retirement plans. They also worked irregular but long hours under nonunion conditions with inadequate protection from work place injustices. Consequently, when COVID-19 touched down in the winter and spring of 2020, large numbers of Black people worked in jobs that placed them in the eye of the storm. They were highly represented among the new "essential workers." They could not stay home, sit in front of the computer, and social distance. Their very survival required that they go out into public and private spaces to drive transportation vehicles, provide caregiving services to the disabled, sick, and elderly; and help to ensure the survival of their communities and the nation.

Despite the provision of such indispensable services, their jobs were by no means secure. They faced recurring layoffs and long periods of unemployment and underemployment. During hard times, unable to pay rent or mortgage payments, eviction and homelessness became an integral part of their lived experience in twenty-first-century America. At the same time, their communities remained targets of lethal policing, mass incarceration, and efforts to turn back the clock on the gains of the Modern Black Freedom Movement. Again, like their forebears, they did not succumb to the overwhelming odds against them. Drawing upon their long legacy of social struggles, they launched a variety of grassroots social movements, most notably Black Lives Matter, and challenged the new postindustrial system of racial inequality and injustice within and beyond the nation's hospitals and other healthcare institutions.

Conclusion

For many contemporary commentators, the twenty-first-century global pandemic, the murder of George Floyd by police officers in Minneapolis, and the substantial economic losses suffered by many in the early years of the pandemic represent the impact of three intersecting pandemics on the health and well-being of Black Americans. As this book has tried to capture, the events and conditions of the 2020s had earlier antecedents in key historical forces: the existence of racist ideology that limited equal access to effective health care (both physical and mental); the struggle to build independent institutions beyond the white gaze and marshal resources to advance both physical and mental wellness; and the emergence of empowerment strategies that evolved in lockstep with shifts in the political economy. Accordingly, COVID-19 and its destructive consequences are a chapter in a longer and more protracted experience that mirror the tightly interwoven histories of African Americans and the nation.

Well into the twentieth century, African Americans encountered entrenched racist ideas, beliefs, and practices within the nation's health care system. Based on the enduring impact of these ideas, the nation's medical establishment routinely neglected the health of Black people—not only through adherence to stereotypes about their immunity to certain diseases that ravaged the lives of Euro-Americans but also through equally damaging beliefs about the presumed "innate" physical weaknesses of the Black body and thus its unusual vulnerability to diseases like tuberculosis during the late nineteenth and early twentieth century.[1] In his pioneering study, *The Philadelphia Negro* (1899), W. E. B. Du Bois called attention to the medical profession's callous attitude toward the health of Black Americans. As Du Bois put it, "The most difficult social problem in the matter of Negro health is the peculiar attitude of the nation toward the well-being of the race. There have, for instance, been few other cases in the history of civilized peoples where human suffering has been viewed with such peculiar indifference." Furthermore, Du Bois continued, when the US Census of 1870 erroneously reported excessively high rates of death among Black people, "Nearly the whole nation seemed delighted [that] . . . the Negroes were dying off rapidly, and the country would soon be well rid of them." Hence, there was presumably no need to expend precious resources on a people "doomed to early extinction."[2]

Nearly a half century later, Swedish economist Gunnar Myrdal summarized a legacy of racial inequality in America's health care system in his classic study, *An American Dilemma* (1944). "Area for area" and "class for class" across the country, he said, "Negroes cannot get the same advantages in the way of preventive [care] and cure of disease that whites can. . . . Discrimination increase Negro sickness and death both directly and indirectly and manifests itself both consciously and unconsciously."[3] Following World War II, in the wake of the Modern Black Freedom Movement and the desegregation of the American medical establishment, scholars, journalists, and public policy analysts soon documented the persistence of racial inequality in the health system despite the collapse of the Jim Crow order. In their detailed study of post–civil rights Black America, *A Common Destiny: Blacks and American Society* (1989), economist Gerald David Jaynes and Robin M. Williams summarized the work of the National Research Council's Committee on the Status of Black Americans. "We write 45 years after Gunnar Myrdal in *An American Dilemma* challenged Americans to bring their racial practices into line with their ideals. Despite clear evidence of progress against each problem [including health among others], Americans face an unfinished agenda: many black Americans remain separated from the mainstream of national life under conditions of great inequality. The American dilemma has not been resolved." The Jaynes and Williams report lamented that "poor blacks, people on Medicaid, and uninsured groups have unmet needs despite expanded health services."[4]

In his foreword to the third edition of Ronald L. Braithwaite, Sandra E. Taylor, and Henrie M. Treadwell's popular text, *Health Issues in the Black Community* (2009), Georges C. Benjamin, past executive director of the American Public Health Association, concluded that the nation's failure to eradicate racial disparities in the health system represented for many "a national tragedy." Indeed, in Benjamin's view, the nation had not only failed to eliminate most health inequities, but "some of them, like the prevalence of HIV and diabetes and the high infant mortality rate in minority communities" had "gotten worse." Moreover, in the same issue, the editors lamented that the third edition "presents a picture of African American health replete with many of the disparities documented in the first two editions. . . . We are still faced with a situation that portends a lowered health status and overall quality of life for the Black community." Mirroring this dismal record, the 2000 US Census reported a life expectancy of 77.8 years for the average Euro-American compared to only 73.1 years for the average African American.[5]

Certain misleading ideas about race and illness continued into twenty-first-century professional medical practices and public health policies. As recently as 2017, in her groundbreaking study on race and the rise of the early American medical profession, historian Rana A. Hogarth noted how medical knowledge also included erroneous racial interpretations of African American disease. Slanted perspectives on race and medicine not only gained widespread attention through the popular media activities of people like Oprah Winfrey and Dr. Oz; they also surfaced among medical professionals writing for more specialized audiences. A significant *body* of scholarship, including references cited by the website of the Centers for Disease Control (CDC), attributed disproportionately high levels of hypertension among African Americans to "the idea of innate racial causes," despite much careful research that underscore the role of "racism and discriminatory practices at the hands of health-care providers or limitations in access to care." As Hogarth puts it, "The allure of racial comparisons in medical discourse has been hard to shake, and it survives, albeit in nuanced forms" to this day.[6] At the turn of the twenty-first century, historian Barbara Jean Fields, the foremost scholar and critic of racial ideology, made the same point. In her words, "The rubric of the hour is race. Though discredited by reputable biologists and geneticists, race has enjoyed a renaissance among historians, sociologists, and literary scholars. They find the concept attractive, or in any case hard to dispense with, and have therefore striven mightily, though in vain to find a basis for it in something other than."[7]

In addition to the ongoing impact of neglect and discrimination by the medical establishment, unhealthy work, housing, and living environments repeatedly reinforced disproportionately high rates of disability, death, and physical and emotional suffering among Black people. From the transatlantic slave trade to North America through the onset of the Civil War, enslaved and free people of color lived and worked in some of the most dangerous and life-threatening environments in the Atlantic world. In relatively rapid succession, their labor fueled the production of the major cash-producing staple crops—tobacco, rice, sugar, and cotton. Each crop imposed its own unique skills, labor demands, and occupational hazards on the enslaved workforce. But a series of overlapping conditions—excessively long hours, close supervision, corporal punishment, and inadequate food, clothing, housing, and medical care—blurred distinctions from crop to crop and exposed Black people to high rates of disease, suffering, and death. To secure regular and uninterrupted labor, guarantee profit margins, and control the workforce, antebellum medical practitioners, slave owners, and employers of free people of color ignored or downplayed the impact of these environmental conditions on both the physical and emotional health of Black people. In their view, mental illness was absent or only temporary or minor phenomena in the lives of African Americans.[8]

The advent of the Civil War and the emancipation of enslaved people dramatically changed the socioeconomic, political, and institutional fortunes of African Americans. For the first time in the nation's history, people of African descent could lay claim to full citizenship rights. Scores of African Americans embarked upon a quest to acquire their own land as the surest foundation for ensuring their freedom, citizenship rights, and health and well-being. But this effort was soon stymied by the reconstruction policies of the federal government as well as the resurgence of ex-confederates in positions of power and influence in the South and across the country. While federal authorities insisted on the negotiation of free labor contracts between formerly enslaved people and former slave owners, such contracts included provisions for food, clothing, and shelter but most often placed medical expenses squarely on the shoulders of freed men and women. The Medical Division of the Freedmen's Bureau provided much-needed medical care for ex-slaves, but it soon closed its doors and left medical needs in the hands of hostile Southern states and municipalities. As such, federal reconstruction policies helped to set the stage for the postbellum rise of the sharecropping system, which exposed African Americans to the sharpest edges of disease and recurring epidemics as the Jim Crow order spread. Tuberculosis also spread rapidly across the country in tandem with the rise of Jim Crow; it claimed the lives of African Americans at three times the rate of their white counterparts.[9]

During the early to mid-twentieth century, African Americans transformed themselves from the nation's most rural to its most urban population. They often celebrated their movement into higher-wage industrial jobs as a "Flight from Egypt," the "New Jerusalem," the "Promised Land," and "Land of Hope," but they soon confronted new challenges to their health and well-being. Racial employment and promotion policies confined them to the most dangerous, arduous, and low-paying jobs as well as the most dilapidated and unhealthy segments of the urban housing market. One popular Detroit automaker spoke for scores of industrial employers when he declared, "We hired them for this hot dirty work and we want them [to stay] there." For his part, one Black autoworker recalled that foremen never considered "a wound as serious enough to go to first aid." In their quest for health care in mainstream medical institutions, they encountered what some medical historians describe as a stiff system of "medical apartheid." In a plethora of jobs in the steel industry, if they survived occupational hazards, "they often contracted occupational diseases such as silicosis, bronchitis, pneumonia, heart disease, and various stomach ailments." [10]

Meanwhile, unlike the antebellum years and earlier, when mental illness among African Americans gained little acknowledgment or attention from the nation's white elites, the postbellum years witnessed growing recognition of mental health issues among newly emancipated people. African Americans gradually gained access to the expanding network of hospitals serving the mentally ill. But their institutional medical treatment unfolded on a racially segregated and unequal basis as the Jim Crow system took hold. Whereas white mental health patients received treatment designed to restore their emotional well-being and return them to their families and communities, Black patients, especially in the South, received work assignments. They cultivated marketable crops and livestock for the financial benefit of the institution. Such work therapy provided little mental health healing and restoration of African Americans to their families and communities.

During the emergence of the Jim Crow order and the spread of the new white supremacist system, medical apartheid gained its most extreme and harshest expression in the infamous 1932 United States Public Health Service Tuskegee Syphilis Study. Without their informed consent, an idea that would only gain widespread currency in the wake of Nazi medical experiments on Jews during World War II, the project recruited poor and working-class Black men for an experiment involving long-term untreated syphilis. [11] In the meantime, beginning gradually during the interwar years, the long medical civil rights movement picked up steam during the 1950s and 1960s, demolished the legal underpinnings of medical apartheid, and opened the door for rising numbers of African Americans to move into the mainstream of the nation's health care system. As the twentieth century came to a close, however, grassroots white opposition to the social welfare state, the collapse of the manufacturing economy, the advent of mass incarceration, and the curtailment of services to poor and working-class Black Americans made them especially vulnerable to the ravages of the AIDS epidemic and later the coronavirus pandemic.

The onset of COVID-19 would also exacerbate and undercut the mental as well as physical health of Black Americans. Assaults on the social welfare system, intertwined with mass incarceration and the growing deinstitutionalization of the mentally ill, resulted in a dramatic transformation of Black mental health care. Across the United States, especially in the South, at the same time that the nation started to desegregate its institutional life in the wake of the US Supreme Court decision in Brown v. Board of Education, industrial-era state hospitals for the mentally ill were increasingly transformed into prisons to house the growing numbers of young Black men and women ensnared in the criminal justice system.

As discussed in this book, when COVID-19 touched down in the winter and spring of 2020, Black people worked in jobs that placed them in the eye of the storm. They were highly represented among the newly discovered "essential workers." They could not stay home, sit in front of the computer, and social distance. Their very survival required that they go out into public and private spaces to drive transportation vehicles; provide caregiving services to the disabled, sick, and elderly; and help to ensure the survival of their communities and the nation. Despite the provision of such indispensable services, their jobs were by no means secure. They faced recurring layoffs and long periods of unemployment and underemployment. Nonunion low-wage work, long hours, no health insurance, minimal protection from workplace injustices, eviction, and even homelessness became integral parts of their lived experience in twenty-first century COVID-era America.[12]

The onslaught of COVID-19 sharply registered in the personal as well as collective experiences of the nation's Black citizenry. On the eve of the pandemic, postindustrial giants like the University of Pittsburgh Medical Center (UPMC) had purchased and consolidated growing numbers of small hospitals and medical centers across the region.[13] Black and white lower-rung health care providers, particularly poor and working-class Black women, worked at the vortex of a new economy dominated by medical and educational institutions. In numerous interviews with historian Gabriel Winant, African Americans vividly described the emergence of unequal working conditions, pay, and treatment in the new health care system. These conditions emerged ahead of COVID-19 but accelerated thereafter. Joyce Henderson described how she joined the health care workforce in the 1970s as a nursing-home employee. She later moved to Presbyterian-University Hospital where she would work for decades, first as a nurse's aide and later as an electrocardiogram (EKG) technician. Still, Henderson emphatically reported how she "felt racialized disrespect from her employer through her entire career" with the firm.

Henderson's experience in the health care sector was by no means static. Along with numerous other Pittsburgh area workers, Henderson described how a major structural transformation engulfed the health care industry as UPMC gained dominance over the field. In her words, work in the health care sector made a dramatic shift from what she described as an earlier (though imperfect) "hospital that cares" to an increasingly austere, insensitive, and demeaning work environment by the turn of the new century. As she put it, "I mean they constantly wanted you to put out, put out, put out, put out, put out. They were like tyrants. And they scrutinized everything that you did. . . . And that's how they did. Somebody left, they didn't replace them. You had to do more, and you had to work more hours, and it was really much."[14] A medical secretary (employed in a UPMC pathology office since 2006) related how the main source of her stress was "her phone constantly ringing, and she cannot miss a call." As Winant summarized this case, "Since everyone else on the unit is overworked too, she finds it difficult to find someone to spell her while she goes to the bathroom. Consequently, every time she needs to pee, she must beg. She believes she has incurred damage to her bladder . . . 'because I was holding my pee so long. I actually peed myself.'"

Housekeeper Janet Dickerson described the toll that the work regimen took on her health: "You're cleaning 30 rooms by yourself . . . you go in wash the bed down, you do all surfaces. You clean the bathroom and you mop that floor and dress that bed and put in the supplies that it needs. You know, to keep it stocked, to stock it, okay . . . I've had two shoulder operations, rotator cuffs and mine just aren't 100% you know to do that all night long." Geneva Davis, a diabetic with high blood pressure and a thyroid condition, described the injustice of working for "a world renowned hospital and there are days when I have to choose between buying food or paying for my medications." Still another UPMC employee held two jobs but still reported no disposable income: "If I do have extra money. I pay it to UPMC—because I have thousands of dollars in healthcare debt." Among male workers, Carl Blue also reported working two jobs for a time within UPMC. "It's very stressful on your body," he said, "but I had to do what I had to do to make it. I did this to make it, to survive, to pay my bills, keep my kids, given the money that's needed to get them what they need for school and things. Just for all of us to be able to survive and eat food, that's why I did it."

Contemporary COVID-era African Americans did not take multiple assaults on their health quietly. As in earlier moments in African American work and medical history, these contemporary postindustrial workers were by no means quiescent. They carried a deep-seated consciousness of their worth and contributions to postindustrial society into the era of the pandemic. In 2015, in testimony before the City of Pittsburgh's Wage Review Committee, health care worker Linda Tabb accented the role of women as drivers of the new health care economy: "This industry is heavily dominated by working mothers, some of them single mothers, all of us doing everything we can to build a good life for ourselves and our families. We are the mothers and the caretakers in the hospitals but it seems like there's no one taking [care] of us or looking out for our wellbeing." Arlene Hill, another health worker, graphically reinforced Tabb's emphasis on the centrality of health care workers in the new political economy of postindustrial Pittsburgh and Western Pennsylvania. "I am an integral part of patient care—from bathing them to emptying bed pans, to being a friendly face when they need one. It's incredibly hard, but I've been at this for thirty years, so I'm obviously not afraid of hard work. I've come to accept the back pain and knee problems I have from lifting patients and being on my feet all day. . . . What I can't accept is the low wages. I am scheduled for thirty six hours a week, but if [I] only worked that much, the only thing I would be able to pay is my rent. There wouldn't be anything for bills, gas, food, or even a new pair of shoes that are on sale." In short, as Winant forcefully concludes, if COVID-19 opened the nation's eyes to the value of low-wage service workers as "essential" employees, these workers themselves had long clearly understood the centrality and value of their own work.

But the era of COVID-19 and the labor and medical rights struggles of Black people are not entirely new phenomena in the nation's history. It is part of a long history of Black health care, class, work, and racial politics reaching back in time before the United States became an independent, though fragile, democratic republic. From the beginning of their residence in North America, in addition to day-to-day efforts to minimize or avoid the most dangerous work assignments as detrimental to their health, African Americans constructed their own informal network of medical care providers, obtained access to their own garden plots, and gradually established their own health, social welfare, and mutual benefit organizations. Perhaps most important, before the start of the Civil War, enslaved and free people of color had built upon their African medical heritage and devised "their own brand of care, complete with special remedies, medical practitioners, and rituals."[15] In the postbellum years, African Americans built upon the health care legacy of their early nineteenth-century forebears.

As the Jim Crow medical establishment expanded and consolidated during the late nineteenth and early twentieth century, African Americans were not content to endure the destructive impact of medical apartheid on their lives. They increased the cultivation of vegetable gardens; expanded the range of medical services available to Black people under the auspices of religious, fraternal, women's clubs, and mutual benefit societies; and developed a vibrant independent Black hospital movement.[16] Similarly, during the era of the Great Migration, they launched a variety of grassroots social movements to counter hazardous work, housing, and living conditions affecting the health and well-being of their families and their communities. Their forceful challenges to the system of medical apartheid reinforced what medical historian and political scientist Alondra Nelson describes as the long medical civil rights movement.[17] Nonetheless, the achievements of the Medical Black Freedom Struggle would not fully hold. Before Black people could genuinely celebrate the passing of medical Jim Crow, the demise of industrial jobs ushered in a new postindustrial regime that continues to unfold today. Still, in the face of COVID-19's disproportionate impact on Black communities, African Americans turned again to their community-based networks and forged creative responses to the pandemic.[18]

Notes

Introduction

1. Chelsey Carter and Ezelle Sanford III, "The Myth of Black Immunity: Racialized Disease during the COVID-19 Pandemic," African American Intellectual History Society (AAIHS), blog post, April 3, 2020; "Coronavirus Outbreak Revives Dangerous Race Myths," *NBC News*, March 19, 2020, transcript; Nick Charles, "Coronavirus Rises to the Forefront for Activists in the Coronavirus Pandemic," *NBC News*, April 10, 2020, online transcript; and Dan Vergano and Kadia Goba, "Why the Coronavirus Is Killing Black Americans at Outsize Rates across the US," *BuzzFeed News*, Science/Coronavirus, April 10, 2020.

2. Georges C. Benjamin, "Foreword," in *Health Issues in the Black Community*, 3rd ed., ed. Ronald L. Braithwaite, Sandra E. Taylor, and Henrie M. Treadwell (San Francisco: Jossey-Bass, 2009), xii; Stephanie E. Smallwood, *Saltwater Slavery: A Middle Passage from Africa to American Diaspora* (Cambridge, MA: Harvard University Press, 2007); Alexander X. Byrd, *Captives and Voyagers: Black Migrants across the Eighteenth-Century British Atlantic World* (Baton Rouge: Louisiana State University Press, 2008); Ira Berlin, *The Making of African America: The Four Great Migrations* (New York: Viking, 2010); Joe William Trotter Jr., *Workers on Arrival: Black Labor in the Making of America* (Oakland: University of California Press, 2019).

3. Samuel A. Cartwright, "Report on the Diseases and Physical Peculiarities of the Negro Race (1851), reprinted in *The Nature of Race in the United States from Jefferson to Genomics*, ed. Evelynn M. Hammonds and Rebecca M. Herzig (Cambridge, MA: MIT Press, 2008), 79–81.

4. Gretchen Long, *Doctoring Freedom: The Politics of African American Medical Care in Slavery and Freedom* (Chapel Hill: The University of North Carolina Press, 2012); Sharla Fett, *Working Cures: Healing, Health, and Power on Southern Slave Plantations* (Chapel Hill: The University of North Carolina Press, 2002); Rana A. Hogarth, *Medicalizing Blackness: Making Racial Difference in the Atlantic World, 1780–1840* (Chapel Hill: The University of North Carolina Press, 2017); Deirdre Cooper Owens, *Medical Bondage: Race, Gender, and the Origins of American Gynecology* (Athens: University of Georgia Press, 2017); Mab Segrest, *Administrations of Lunacy: Racism and the Haunting of American Psychiatry at the Milledgeville Asylum* (New York: The New Press, 2020), xvi (Morrison quote).

5. Jim Downs, *Sick from Freedom: African-American Illness and Suffering during the Civil War and Reconstruction* (New York: Oxford University Press, 2012); Steven Hahn, *A Nation under Our Feet: Black Political Struggles in the Rural South from Slavery to the Great Migration* (Cambridge, MA: Harvard University Press, 2003); David McBride, *Caring for Equality: A History of African American Health and Healthcare* (Lanham, MD: Rowman

and Littlefield, 2018); W. Michael Byrd and Linda Clayton, *An American Health Dilemma: A Medical History African Americans and the Problem of Race, Beginnings to 1900* (New York: Routledge, 2000); Margaret Humphreys, *Intensely Human: The Health of the Black Soldier in the American Civil War* (Baltimore: Johns Hopkins University Press, 2008); Vanessa Northington Gamble, *Making Place for Ourselves: The Black Hospital Movement, 1920–1945* (New York: Oxford University Press, 1995).

6. Leah Platt Boustan, *Competition in the Promised Land: Black Migrants in Northern Cities and Labor Markets* (Princeton, NJ: Princeton University Press, 2017); James N. Gregory, *The Southern Diaspora: How the Great Migrations of Black and White Southerners Transformed America* (Chapel Hill: The University of North Carolina Press, 2005); Carol Marks, *Farewell—We're Good and Gone: The Great Black Migration* (Bloomington: Indiana University Press, 1989); Isabel Wilkerson, *The Warmth of Other Suns: The Epic Story of America's Great Migration* (New York: Random House, 2010); Berlin, *The Making of African America*; Steven A. Reich, *A Working People: A History of African American Workers Since Emancipation* (Lanham, MD: Rowman and Littlefield, 2013).

7. Gabriel Winant, *The Next Shift: The Fall of Industry and the Rise of Health Care in Rust Belt America* (Cambridge, MA: Harvard University Press, 2021); Michael L. Bagshaw and Robert H. Schnorbus, "The Local Labor-Market Response to a Plant Shutdown," Federal Reserve Bank of Cleveland, January 1980; Stuart Auerbach, "US Steel Set to Close Plants, End 15,000 Jobs," *Washington Post*, December 28, 1983; Reich, *A Working People*; Reynolds Farley, Sheldon Danziger, and Harry J. Holzer, *Detroit Divided: A Volume in the Multi-City Study of Urban* Inequality (New York: Russell Sage Foundation, 2000); Lawrence D. Bobo, Melvin L. Oliver, James H. Johnson Jr., and Abel Valenzuela Jr., *The Prismatic Metropolis: Inequality in Los Angeles* (New York: Russell Sage Foundation, 2000); Robert H. Zieger, *For Jobs and Freedom: Race and Labor in America Since 1865* (Lexington: University Press of Kentucky, 2007); David McBride, *From TB to AIDS: Epidemics among Urban Blacks since 1900* (Albany: State University of New York Press, 1991). Note: I employ the terms "postindustrial" and "digital" age interchangeably.

8. R. S. Evans, "Electronic Health Records: Then, Now, and in the Future," International Academy of Health Sciences Informatics (IAHS), *Yearbook of Medical Informatics*, supp. 1 (May 20, 2016): S48–S6; Bridget Balch, "Making Medicine Personal: Moving Away from a One-Size Fits All Approach to Health Care," Association of American Medical Colleges, *AAMCNews*, February 22, 2024.

Chapter One

1. Ira Berlin, *The Making of African America: Four Great Migrations* (New York: Viking, 2010), 14–15; Stephanie E. Smallwood, *Saltwater Slavery: A Middle Passage from Africa to American Diaspora* (Cambridge, MA: Harvard University Press, 2007); Alexander X. Byrd, *Captives and Voyagers: Black Migrants across the Eighteenth-Century British Atlantic World* (Baton Rouge: Louisiana State University Press, 2008); Marcus Rediker, *The Slave Ship: A Human History* (New York: Viking, 2007); Philip D. Morgan, *Slave Counterpoint: Black Culture in the Eighteenth-Century Chesapeake and Lowcountry* (Chapel Hill: The University of North Carolina Press, 1998); Todd L. Savitt, *Medicine and*

Slavery: The Diseases and Health Care of Blacks in Antebellum Virginia (Urbana: University of Illinois Press, 1978); Peter Wood, Black Majority: Negroes in Colonial South Carolina from 1670 through the Stono Rebellion (New York: W. W. Norton, 1974).

2. Rana A. Hogarth, Medicalizing Blackness: Making Racial Difference in the Atlantic World, 1780-1840 (Chapel Hill: The University of North Carolina Press, 2017); Gretchen Long, Doctoring Freedom: The Politics of African American Medical Care in Slavery and Freedom (Chapel Hill: The University of North Carolina Press, 2012); Mab Segrest, Administrations of Lunacy: Racism and the Haunting of American Psychiatry at the Milledgeville Asylum (New York: The New Press, 2020); Stephen C. Kenny, "The Development of Medical Museums in the Antebellum American South: Slave Bodies in Networks of Anatomical Exchange," Bulletin of the History of Medicine 87 (Spring 2013): 32-62; Sharla Fett, Working Cures: Healing, Health, and Power on Southern Slave Plantations (Chapel Hill: The University of North Carolina Press, 2002); Deirdre Cooper Owens, Medical Bondage: Race, Gender, and the Origins of American Gynecology (Athens: University of Georgia Press, 2017); Daina Ramey Berry, The Price for Their Pound of Flesh: The Value of the Enslaved, from Womb to Grave, in the Building of the Nation (Boston: Beacon Press, 2017); Edward Baptist, The Half Has Never Been Told: Slavery and the Making of American Capitalism (New York: Basic Books, 2014); Walter Johnson, River of Dark Dreams: Slavery and Empire in the Cotton Kingdom (Cambridge, MA: The Belknap Press of Harvard University, 2013); Paul Starr, The Social Transformation of American Medicine: The Rise of a Sovereign Profession and the Making of a Vast Industry (New York: Basic Books, 1982); W. Michael Byrd and Linda Clayton, An American Health Dilemma: A Medical History of African Americans and the Problem of Race, Beginnings to 1900 (New York: Routledge, 2000); Harriet Washington, Medical Apartheid: The Dark History of Medical Experimentation on Black Americans from Colonial Times (New York: Doubleday, 2006); Jacqueline Jones, American Work: Four Centuries of Black and White Labor (New York: W. W. Norton, 1998); David McBride, Caring for Equality: A History of African American Health and Healthcare (Lanham, MD: Rowman and Littlefield, 2018); Evelyn M. Hammonds and Rebecca M. Herzig, eds., The Nature of Difference: Science of Race in the United States from Jefferson to Genomics (Cambridge, MA: MIT Press, 2008).

3. Hogarth, Medicalizing Blackness, 1-13; Starr, The Social Transformation of American Medicine, 3.

4. Quoted in Savitt, Medicine and Slavery, 22, 8-21, 219-21, 240-46; Mariola Espinosa, "The Question of Racial Immunity to Yellow Fever in History and Historiography," Social Science History 38 (Winter 2014): 437-53; Wood, Black Majority, xviii; Jim Downs, Sick from Freedom: African American Illness and Suffering during the Civil War and Reconstruction (New York: Oxford University Press, 2021), 34.

5. Hogarth, Medicalizing Blackness, 19.

6. Byrd and Clayton, An American Health Dilemma, 63, 220-21, 301; Starr, The Social Transformation of American Medicine, 3.

7. Long, Doctoring Freedom, 11.

8. Segrest, Administrations of Lunacy, 35-36.

9. Segrest, 35-36.

10. Segrest, 35-36.

11. Savitt, Medicine and Slavery, 248-49.

12. Savitt, 248–49; Segrest, *Administrations of Lunacy*, 37.

13. Segrest, 37.

14. Londa Schiebinger, "Medical Experimentation and Race in the Eighteenth-Century Atlantic World," *Social History of Medicine* 26 (2013): 364–82.

15. Kenny, "The Development of Medical Museums in the Antebellum American South."

16. Byrd and Clayton, *An American Health Dilemma, to 1900*, 271–75.

17. Owens, *Medical Bondage*, 1–14; Washington, *Medical Apartheid*, quote, 2.

18. Owens, *Medical Bondage*, 89–107; Washington, *Medical Apartheid*, 2, 4, 52–53.

19. Quoted in Berry, *The Price for Their Pound of Flesh*, 167; Walter Johnson, *Soul by Soul: Life Inside the Antebellum Slave Market* (Cambridge, MA: Harvard University Press, 1999), 102–4.

20. Johnson, *Soul by Soul*, 120–21.

21. Berry, *The Price for Their Pound of Flesh*, 7; Robert L. Blakely and Judith M. Harrington, eds., *Bones in the Basement: Postmortem Racism in Nineteenth-Century Medical Training* (Washington, DC: Smithsonian Institution Press, 1997), 162–63, 206–7.

22. Blakely and Harrington, "Grave Consequences: The Opportunistic Procurement of Cadavers at the Medical College of Georgia," quoted in Blakely and Harrington, *Bones in the Basement*, 163.

23. Savitt, *Medicine and Slavery*, 292.

24. Berry, *The Price for Their Pound of Flesh*, 177.

25. Washington, *Medical Apartheid*, 126.

26. Berry, *The Price for Their Pound of Flesh*, 169.

27. Fett, *Working Cures*, 7, 11, 25–27.

28. Quoted in Fett, 15, 18.

29. Hogarth, *Medicalizing Blackness*, 159–60.

30. Hogarth, 66, 170, 172.

31. Vanessa Northington Gamble, *Making Place for Ourselves: The Black Hospital Movement, 1920–1945* (New York: Oxford University Press, 1995), 4–5; Savitt (*Medicine and Slavery*, 194, 209–10) notes that some free people of color paid a fee to gain access to health care service.

32. Morgan, *Slave Counterpoint*, 169; Ira Berlin, *Many Thousands Gone: The First Two Centuries of Slavery in North America* (Cambridge: Belknap Press, 1998), 116–17.

33. Morgan, *Slave Counterpoint*, 168.

34. Savitt, *Medicine and Slavery*, 107–8.

35. Morgan, *Slave Counterpoint*, 147–49.

36. Berlin, *Many Thousands Gone*, 146; Morgan, *Slave Counterpoint*, 149, 156–57.

37. Morgan, *Slave Counterpoint*, 149.

38. Berlin, *Many Thousands Gone*, 146; quoted in Morgan, *Slave Counterpoint*, 149, 156–57.

39. Morgan, *Slave Counterpoint*, 149.

40. Quoted in Wood, *Black Majority*, 78; Byrd and Clayton, *An American Health Dilemma*, 225–26.

41. Wood, *Black Majority*, 151–53.

42. Daniel H. Usner Jr., "From African Captivity to American Slavery: The Introduction of Black Laborers to Colonial Louisiana," *Louisiana History* 20 (1979): 38–47;
D. H. Usner Jr., *Indians, Settlers, and Slaves in an Exchange Economy: The Lower Mississippi Valley before 1783* (Chapel Hill: The University of North Carolina Press, 1992),
31–34, 54–56; Gwendolyn Midlo Hall, *Africans in Colonial Louisiana: The Development
of Afro-Creole Culture in the Eighteenth Century* (Baton Rouge: Louisiana State University Press, 1992), 126–27, 179.

43. Berlin, *Many Thousands Gone*, 86, 340–41, 343; Baptist, *The Half Has Never Been
Told*, 56; Rebecca Scott, *Degrees of Freedom: Louisiana and Cuba after Slavery* (Cambridge, MA: Harvard University Press, 2005), 12.

44. Roderick A. McDonald, "Independent Economic Production by Slaves on Antebellum Louisiana Sugar Plantations," in Ira Berlin and Philip D. Morgan, *Cultivation and Culture: Labor and the Shaping of Slave Life in the Americas* (Charlottesville:
University of Virginia Press, 1993), 207; Usner, "From African Captivity to American Slavery," 28, 33; R. Scott, *Degrees of Freedom*, 12.

45. Hamilton as cited in McDonald, "Independent Economic Production by Slaves
on Antebellum Louisiana Sugar Plantations," 277–78.

46. McDonald, "Independent Economic Production by Slaves on Antebellum Louisiana Sugar Plantations," 277.

47. Usner, "From African Captivity to American Slavery," 38.

48. Usner, 33.

49. Adam Rothman, *Slave Country: American Expansion and the Origins of the Deep
South* (Cambridge, MA: Harvard University Press, 2005), 77.

50. Rothman, *Slave Country*, 190.

51. All quotes from Fett, *Working Cures*, 25.

52. Steven F. Miller, "Plantation Labor Organization and Slav Life on the Cotton
Frontier: The Alabama-Mississippi Black Belt, 1815–1840," in Berlin and Morgan,
Cultivation and Culture, 158; Berlin, *Many Thousands Gone*, 345.

53. William Kauffman Scarborough, *The Overseer: Plantation Management in the Old
South* (Athens: University of Georgia Press, 1984), 25–29.

54. Savitt, *Medicine and Slavery*, 111–12; Baptist, *The Half Has Never Been Told*, 120–21.

55. Baptist, *The Half Has Never Been Told*, quotes, 121.

56. Deborah Gray White, *Ar'n't I a Woman?: Female Slaves in the Plantation South*
(New York: W. W. Norton, 1985), 33.

57. Byrd and Clayton, *An American Health Dilemma, to 1900*, 226; Savitt, *Medicine
and Slavery*, 90–93.

58. This and the following paragraph is based on Savitt, *Medicine and Slavery*, 52–53,
54–80, 104. Also see Byrd and Clayton, *An American Health Dilemma*, 227.

59. Savitt, *Medicine and Slavery*, 49–50, 57–73 (especially 57–58), 60–61, 80–82,
106–10, 115–29, 226–40; Richard C. Wade, *Slavery in the Cities: The South, 1820-1860*
(London: Oxford University Press, 1964), 33–43; Ronald L. Lewis, *Coal, Iron, and
Slaves: Industrial Slavery in Maryland and Virginia, 1715-1865* (Westport, CT.: Green-
wood Press, 1979), 154–55; T. Stephen Whitman, *The Price of Freedom: Slavery and
Manumission in Baltimore and Early National Maryland* (Lexington: University Press of
Kentucky, 1997), 37–39, 48, 53.

60. Savitt, *Medicine and Slavery*, 60.

61. Wade, *Slavery in the Cities*, 33–43; Lewis, *Coal, Iron, and Slaves*, 154–55; Whitman, *The Price of Freedom*, 37–39, 48, 53;. Also, see Savitt, *Medicine and Slavery*, 80–82, 106–10, 226–40.

62. Catherine Adams and Elizabeth H. Pleck, *Love of Freedom: Black Women in Colonial and Revolutionary New England* (New York: Oxford University Press, 2010), 32–35, quote, 34; Seth Rockman, *Scraping By: Wage Labor, Slavery, and Survival in Early Baltimore* (Baltimore: Johns Hopkins University Press, 2009), 100–103; Jane E. Dabel, *A Respectable Woman: The Public Roles of African American Women in Nineteenth-Century New York* (New York: New York University Press, 2008), 6–7, 15–16, 78, 82–83; Wilma King, *The Essence of Liberty: Free Black Women during the Slave Era* (Columbia: University of Missouri Press, 2006), 61–72; Suzanne Lebsock, *The Free Women of Petersburg: Status and Culture in a Southern Town, 1784–1860* (New York: Norton, 1984), 97–98; Cynthia M. Kennedy, *Braided Relations, Entwined Lives: The Women of Charleston's Urban Slave Society* (Bloomington: Indiana University Press, 2005), 66.

63. Adams and Pleck, *Love of Freedom*, 32–35, 37; Kennedy, *Braided Relations, Entwined Lives*, 120–21; Dabel, *A Respectable Woman*, 6–7, 15–16, 78, 82–83; Lebsock, *The Free Women of Petersburg*, 97–98; King, *The Essence of Liberty*, 66–69; Rockman, *Scraping By*, 129–30.

64. Savitt, *Medicine and Slavery*, 80.

65. Dorceta E. Taylor, *The Environment and the People in American Cities, 1600s–1900s* (Durham, NC: Duke University Press, 2009), 669–70; Byrd and Clayton, *An American Health Dilemma, to 1900*, 237; Evelynn Hammonds, "Healthcare Disparities: A Long View," *The HistoryMakers Newsletter*, May 8, 2020. For an interview with Evelynn Hammonds, see Isaac Chotiner, "How Racism Is Shaping the Coronavirus Pandemic," *The New Yorker*, May 7, 2020.

66. Taylor, *The Environment and the People*, quote, 70. The next two paragraphs are also based on Taylor, 70, 75–76, 83, 85. For information on Blacks during Philadelphia's yellow fever epidemic of 1793, also see Taylor, 70–75.

67. Quotes are from Wood, *Black Majority*, xviii; Savitt, *Medicine and Slavery*, 18–21.

68. Taylor, *The Environment and the People*, 69–72, 76, 81.

69. Gamble, *Making Place for Ourselves*, 4–5. Savitt notes that some free people of color paid a fee to gain access to health care service; see Savitt, *Medicine and Slavery*, 194, 209–10.

70. Gamble, *Making Place for Ourselves*, 6; W. Michael Byrd and Linda A. Clayton, *An American Health Dilemma: A Medical History of African Americans and the Problem of Race, Beginnings to 1900* (New York: Routledge, 2000), 212–13, 233; Byrd and Clayton, *An American Health Dilemma, 1900–2000: Race, Medicine, and Health Care in the United States, 1900–2000* (New York: Routledge, 2002), xv. Early medical facilities in the North and South that served Blacks on a segregated basis, if at all, included Philadelphia's Almshouse (1731); New York City's Bellevue (1737); the Pennsylvania Hospital (1751); the New York Hospital (1791); and the New Orleans Charity Hospital (1737).

71. Fett, *Working Cures*, 1.

72. McBride, *Caring for Equality*, 11.

73. Savitt, *Medicine and Slavery*, 149–50; Fett, *Working Cures*, 2; Byrd and Clayton, *An American Health Dilemma, to 1900*, 240.

74. Fett, *Working Cures*, 15, 18, 20, 34, 36; Savitt, *Medicine and Slavery*, 149–50.

75. Fett, *Working Cures*, 20, 34, 36, 37, 41, 51.

76. Quoted in *Usner*, "From African Captivity to American Slavery," 33; Byrd and Clayton, *An American Health Dilemma*, 240.

77. Byrd and Clayton, *An American Health Dilemma, to 1900*, 232, 240–41; Savitt, *Medicine and Slavery*, 175–76.

78. Savitt, *Medicine and Slavery*, 181–82, 186.

79. Savitt, 183.

80. Owens, *Medical Bondage*, 1–2, 111–14; Long, *Doctoring Freedom*, 122.

81. Owens, *Medical Bondage*, 1–2; Darlene Clark Hine, *Black Women in White: Racial Conflict and Cooperation in the Nursing Profession, 1890–1950* (Bloomington: Indiana University Press, 1989), 3–4; Savitt, *Medicine and Slavery*, 180–81.

82. Roi Ottley and William J. Weatherby, *The Negro in New York: An Informal Social History* (New York: New York Public Library and Oceana Publications, 1967), 12; Byrd and Clayton, *An American Health Dilemma, to 1900*, 241.

83. Washington, *Medical Apartheid*, 148, 150; Byrd and Clayton, *An American Health Dilemma*, 305.

84. Washington, 146–47.

85. Byrd and Clayton, *An American Health Dilemma*, 307–9, 312–13.

86. For all quotes on slaves' access to land and property, see Loren L. Schweninger, *Black Property Owners in the South, 1790–1915* (Urbana: University of Illinois Press, 1990), 13–14, 30–31; Juliet E. K. Walker, *The History of Black Business in America: Capitalism, Race, Entrepreneurship, Vol. 1, to 1865*, 2nd ed. (Chapel Hill: The University of North Carolina Press, 2009), 81–82; Robert Olwell, *Masters, Slaves, and Subjects: South Carolina Low Country, 1740–1790* (Ithaca, NY: Cornell University Press, 1998), 149–50.

87. Savitt, *Medicine and Slavery*, 95–96; Byrd and Clayton, *An American Health Dilemma*, 225–26.

88. Theda Skocpol, Ariane Liazos, and Marshall Ganz, *What a Mighty Power We Can Be: African American Fraternal Groups and the Struggle for Racial Equality* (Princeton, NJ: Princeton University Press, 2006), 2–3, 34; Joe W. Trotter, "African American Fraternal Associations in American History: An Introduction," and Theda Skocpol and Jennifer L. Oser, "Organization Despite Adversity: The Origins and Development of African American Fraternal Associations," special issue, *Social Science History* 28, no. 3 (Fall 2004), 355–66, 373–87.

89. Christopher Phillips, *Freedom's Port: The African American Community of Baltimore, 1790–1860* (Urbana: University of Illinois Press, 1997), 78, 170–71, 202; Chris M. Asch and George D. Musgrove, *Chocolate City: A History of Race and Democracy in the Nation's Capital* (Chapel Hill: The University of North Carolina Press, 2017), 60–61; Ira Berlin, *Slaves without Masters: The Free Negro in the Antebellum South* (New York: Oxford University Press, 1974), 234–41; Leonard P. Curry, *The Free Black Urban America, 1900–1850: The Shadow of the Dream* (Chicago: University of Chicago Press, 1981), 25–36; Philip S. Foner, *Organized Labor and the Black Worker, 1619–1973* (New York: Praeger Publishers,

1974), 10–11; Philip Foner and Ronald Lewis, ed., *The Black Worker to 1869, Vol. 1* (Philadelphia: Temple University Press, 1978), 236–41, 245–46.

90. Whittington B. Johnson, *Black Savannah, 1788-1864* (Fayetteville: University of Arkansas Press, 1996), 121; John Blassingame, *Black New Orleans, 1865-1880* (Chicago: University of Chicago Press, 1973), 11: Bernard E. Powers Jr., *Black Charlestonians: A Social History, 1822-1885* (Fayetteville: University of Arkansas Press, 1994), 51. Despite the Brown Fellowship efforts to reach poor and free people of color, dark-skinned free people of color took steps to organize for their own social welfare with the creation of the Society of Dark Men or the Humane Brotherhood. (Powers, *Black Charlestonians*, 52).

91. See the innovative dissertation and book in progress by Aishah Scott, "Respectability Can't Save You: The Aids Epidemic in Black America" (PhD diss., Stony Brook University, 2019), 44; Savitt, *Medicine and Slavery*, 18, 219–21, 240–46.

92. Gary Nash, *Forging Freedom: The Formation of Philadelphia's Black Community, 1720-1840* (Cambridge, MA: Harvard University Press, 1988), 121–25, 273–77; Julie Winch, *Philadelphia's Black Elite: Activism, Accommodation, and the Struggle for Autonomy, 1787-1848* (Philadelphia: Temple University Press, 1988), 15–17; James Oliver Horton and Lois E. Horton, *In Hope of Liberty: Culture, Community, and Protest among Northern Free Blacks, 1700-1860* (New York: Oxford University Press, 1997), 90–92; Richard S. Newman, *Freedom's Prophet: Bishop Richard Allen, the A. M. E. Church, and the Black Founding Fathers* (New York: New York University Press, 2008), 84–95; Scott, "Respectability Can't Save You," quotes, 45.

Chapter Two

1. Mab Segrest, *Administrations of Lunacy: Racism and the Haunting of American Psychiatry at the Milledgeville Asylum* (New York: New Press, 2020), quote, 113.

2. Jim Downs, *Sick from Freedom: African-American Illness and Suffering during the Civil War and Reconstruction* (New York: Oxford University Press, 2012), 103; Steven Hahn, *A Nation under Our Feet: Black Political Struggles in the Rural South from Slavery to the Great Migration* (Cambridge, MA: Harvard University Press, 2003); David McBride, *Caring for Equality: A History of African American Health and Healthcare* (Lanham, MD: Rowman and Littlefield, 2018); W. Michael Byrd and Linda Clayton, *An American Health Dilemma: A Medical History African Americans and the Problem of Race, Beginnings to 1900* (New York: Routledge, 2000).

3. McBride, *Caring for Equality*, 18.

4. Downs, *Sick from Freedom*, 4.

5. Downs, 4.

6. See Edda L. Fields-Black, *Combee: Harriet Tubman, the Combahee River Raid, and Black Freedom during the Civil War* (New York: Oxford University Press, 2024); Tiya Miles, *Night Flyer: Harriet Tubman and the Faith Dreams of a Free People* (New York: Penguin Press, 2024).

7. Margaret Humphreys, *Intensely Human: The Health of the Black Soldier in the American Civil War* (Baltimore: Johns Hopkins University Press, 2008), 3, 6, 74, 79; McBride, *Caring for Equality*, 31–33.

8. Cited in Margaret Humphreys, *Malaria: Poverty, Race, and Public Health* (Baltimore: Johns Hopkins University Press, 2001), 45–50, and Humphreys, *Intensely Human*, 11; "Statistics on the Civil War and Medicine," Ohio State University, E-History, https://ehistory.osu.edu/exhibitions/cwsurgeon/cwsurgeon/statistics.

9. Humphreys, *Intensely Human*, 9–12.

10. Herbert M. Morais, *The History of the Negro in Medicine: International Library of Negro Life and History* (New York: Publishers Company, 1967), 49; Elizabeth Rauh Bethel, *Promiseland: A Century of Life in a Negro Community* (Philadelphia: Temple University Press, 1981), 25–26; Harriet A. Washington, *Medical Apartheid: The Dark History of Medical Experimentation on Black Americans from Colonial Times to the Present* (New York: Doubleday, 2006), 152.

11. Downs, *Sick from Freedom*, 3–4; Byrd and Clayton, *An American Health Dilemma*, quotes, 322, 349.

12. Vanessa Northington Gamble, *Making Place for Ourselves: The Black Hospital Movement, 1920–1945* (New York: Oxford University Press, 1995), 12; Downs, *Sick from Freedom*, 103.

13. McBride, *Caring for Equality*, 19–20; Washington, *Medical Apartheid*, 151.

14. Howard N. Rabinowitz, *Race Relations in the Urban South, 1865–1890* (New York: Oxford University Press, 1978), 131.

15. Leon Litwack, *Been in the Storm So Long: The Aftermath of Slavery* (1979; pb. New York: Vintage Books, 1980), 396–97.

16. For later discussions of "stress" in Black medical history, see Ronald L. Braithwaite, Sandra E. Taylor, and Henrie M. Treadwell, eds., *Health Issues in the Black Community*, 3rd ed. (San Francisco: Jossey-Bass, 2009), esp. 35–95, for the specialized essays on the health status of African American children, adolescents, men, and women. See also Nancy Krieger, Anna Kosheleva, Pamela D. Waterman, Jarvis T. Chen, and Karestan Koenen, "Racial Discrimination, Psychological Distress, and Self-Rated Health among US-Born and Foreign-Born Black Americans," *American Journal of Public Health* 101, no. 9 (2011): 1704–13; and David R. William, Yan Yu, James S. Jackson, and Norman B. Anderson, "Racial Differences in Physical and Mental Health: Socio-Economic Status, Stress and Discrimination," *Journal of Health Psychology* 2, no. 3 (1997): 335–51.

17. Segrest, *Administrations of Lunacy*, 112.

18. Segrest, quote, 146.

19. Paul Starr, *The Social Transformation of American Medicine: The Rise of a Sovereign Profession and the Making of a Vast Industry* (New York: Basic Books, 1982), 137–38.

20. Lundy Braun, *Breathing Race into the Machine: The Surprising Career of the Spirometer from Plantation to Genetics* (Minneapolis: University of Minnesota Press, 2014), xxiii, 31–47; Humphreys, *Intensely Human*, 50–52; Byrd and Clayton, *An American Health Dilemma*, 338–39.

21. Humphreys, *Intensely Human*, 51; McBride, *Caring for Equality*, 10, 14–15; David McBride, *From TB to AIDS: Epidemics among Urban Blacks since 1900* (Albany: State University of New York Press, 1991), 15.

22. Evelyn M. Hammonds and Rebecca M. Herzig, eds., *The Nature of Difference: Sciences of Race in the United States from Jefferson to Genomics* (Cambridge, MA: MIT Press, 2008), 107–9.

23. Hammonds and Herzig; Byrd and Clayton, *An American Health Dilemma*, 77–78; McBride, *From TB to AIDS*, 16.

24. For both D. D. Quillian and T. W. Murray quotes, see McBride, *From TB to AIDS*, 18–20; and Washington, *Medical Apartheid*, 160.

25. John S. Haller Jr., *Outcasts from Evolution: Scientific Attitudes of Racial Inferiority, 1859-1900* (Urbana: University of Illinois Press, 1971), cited in Byrd and Clayton, *An American Health Dilemma*, 412. For insight into the way these ideas would fuel the emergence of the eugenics movement in England and the United States, see Michael Yudell, *Race Unmasked: Biology and Race in the 20th Century* (New York: Columbia University Press, 2014).

26. Downs, *Sick from Freedom*, 15.

27. Gamble, *Making Place for Ourselves*, 12; Downs, *Sick from Freedom*, 103.

28. Tera W. Hunter, *To 'Joy My Freedom: Southern Black Women's Lives and Labors after the Civil War* (Cambridge, MA: Harvard University Press, 1997), chap. 4, "Tuberculosis as the 'Negro Servants' Disease"; and Edward H. Beardsley, *A History of Neglect: Health Care for Blacks and Mill Workers in the Twentieth-Century South* (Knoxville: University of Tennessee Press, 1987), 13–26.

29. Gamble, *Making Place for Ourselves*, 7, 13 (on fear of experimentation); Hunter, *To 'Joy My Freedom*, 199–200; Byrd and Clayton, *An American Health Dilemma*, 14.

30. Starr, *The Social Transformation of Medicine*, 157–58.

31. Starr, 172–73.

32. Downs, *Sick from Freedom*, 8.

33. Downs, 128–29.

34. Gretchen Long, *Doctoring Freedom: The Politics of African American Medical Care in Slavery and Emancipation* (Chapel Hill: The University of North Carolina Press, 2012), 141.

35. Robert H. Zieger, *For Jobs and Freedom: Race and Labor in America Since 1865* (Lexington: University Press of Kentucky, 2007), quote, 10; David E. Bernstein, *Only One Place of Redress: African Americans, Labor Regulations, and the Courts from Reconstruction to the New Deal* (Durham: Duke University Press, 2001), 10–16; Edward Royce, *The Origins of Southern Sharecropping* (Philadelphia: Temple University Press, 1993), 115–18.

36. Litwack, *Been in the Storm*, 337.

37. Milton Meltzer, ed., *In Their Own Words: A History of the American Negro, 1865–1916* (New York: Thomas Y. Crowell Company, 1965), 135–46.

38. Donald Nieman, *Promises to Keep: African-Americans and the Constitutional Order, 1776-Present* (New York: Oxford University Press, 1991), 73; Steven A. Reich, *A Working People: A History of African American Workers since Emancipation* (Lanham, MD: Rowman and Littlefield, 2013), 21–22, 24–26, 28–31; Bernstein, *Only One Place of Redress*, 8–10; Gerald David Jaynes, *Branches Without Roots: Genesis of the Black Working Class in the American South, 1862-1882* (New York: Oxford University Press, 1986), 153–57; Eric Foner, *Reconstruction: America's Unfinished Revolution, 1863-1877* (New York: Harper and Row, 1988), 373; Gamble, *Making Place for Ourselves*, 7; Rabinowitz, *Race Relations in the Urban South*, 133; Royce, *The Origins of Southern Sharecropping*, 181–84, 214–19; William H. Harris, *The Harder We Run: Black Workers since the Civil War* (New York: Oxford University Press, 1982), 10–13.

39. Jacqueline Jones, *A Dreadful Deceit: The Myth of Race from the Colonial Era to Obama's America* (New York: Basic Books, 2013), 198.

40. Reich, *A Working People*, 38.

41. Pete Daniel, *Breaking the Land: The Transformation of Cotton, Tobacco, and Rice Cultures since 1880* (Urbana: University of Illinois Press, 1985), quote, 14–15.

42. Jaynes, *Branches Without Roots*, 148–49; Julie Saville, *The Work of Reconstruction: From Slave to Wage Laborer in South Carolina, 1860-1870* (Cambridge: Cambridge University Press, 1996), 125–30; Leslie A. Schwalm, *A Hard Fight for We: Women's Transition from Slavery to Freedom* (Urbana: University of Illinois Press, 1997), 226–27, 230–31; Florette Henri, *Black Migration: Movement North, 1900-1920* (Garden City: Anchor Press/ Doubleday, 1975), 27–28; Jacqueline Jones, *Dispossessed: America's Underclass from the Civil War to the Present* (New York: Basic Books, 1992), 77; Daniel M. Johnson and Rex R. Campbell, *Black Migration in America: A Social Demographic History* (Durham: Duke University Press, 1981), 70; Nell Irvin Painter, *Exodusters: Black Migration to Kansas after Reconstruction* (Lawrence: University of Kansas, 1976), 54–81; Gunnar Myrdal, *An American Dilemma: The Negro Problem and Modern Democracy, Volume I* (New York: Pantheon Books, 1962 reprint), 234–35.

43. Rabinowitz, *Race Relations in the Urban South*, 97–101; Earl Lewis, *In Their Own Interests: Race, Class, and Power in Twentieth-Century Norfolk, Virginia* (Berkeley: University of California Press, 1991); James Borchert, *Alley Life in Washington: Family, Community, Religion, and Folklife in the City, 1850-1970* (Urbana: University of Illinois Press, 1980), 3–6; Joe William Trotter Jr., *The African American Experience* (Boston: Houghton Mifflin Company, 2001), 322.

44. Trotter, *The African American Experience*, quote, 325–26.

45. Rabinowitz, *Race Relations in the Urban South*, 134.

46. See Krieger et al., "Racial Discrimination, Psychological Distress, and Self-Rated Health Among US-Born and Foreign-Born Black Americans."

47. Nan Elizabeth Woodruff, *American Congo: The African American Freedom Struggle in the Delta* (Cambridge, MA: Harvard University Press, 2003), 22–23; Susan L. Smith, *Sick and Tired of Being Sick and Tired: Black Women's Health Activism in America, 1890-1950* (Philadelphia: University of Pennsylvania Press, 1995), chaps. 1 and 2; James C. Cobb, *The Most Southern Place on Earth: The Mississippi Delta and the Roots of Regional Identity* (New York: Oxford University Press, 1992), 82. Of note is the case of Arkansas and the life of Delta Black landowner Scott Bond (Woodruff, 12–13); in the Mississippi Delta, Black landownership dropped from 7.3 percent in 1900 to 3.0 percent in 1910 (Cobb, 82).

48. Gilbert Fite, *Cotton Fields No More: Southern Agriculture, 1865-1980* (Lexington: University Press of Kentucky, 1984), 35; Bethel, *Promiseland*, 72.

49. Jones, *A Dreadful Deceit*, 204–5.

50. Reich, *A Working People*, 22–31.

51. Jacqueline Jones, *Labor of Love, Labor of Sorrow: Black Women, Work, and the Family, from Slavery to the Present* (New York: Basic Books, 1985), 137–41.

52. Reich, *A Working People*, 25–28.

53. Reich, *A Working People*, 28–31; Schwalm, *A Hard Fight for We*, 147–53, 161–63.

54. Jones, *Labor of Love, Labor of Sorrow*, 59; Schwalm, *A Hard Fight for We*, 206.

55. Lewis, *In Their Own Interests*, xxx; Joe William Trotter Jr., *Coal, Class, and Color: Blacks in Southern West Virginia, 1915-32* (Urbana: University of Illinois Press, 1990), xxx.

56. David Rosner and Gerald Markowitz, eds., *Dying for Work: Workers' Safety and Health in Twentieth-Century America* (Bloomington: Indiana University Press, 1989), 37; Reich, *A Working People*, 43; Rabinowitz, *Race Relations in the Urban South*, 63; Bernard E. Powers Jr., *Black Charlestonians: A Social History, 1822-1885* (Fayetteville: University of Arkansas Press, 1994), 105, 126, 133, 168-69; Allen H. Stokes Jr., "Black and White Labor and the Development of the Southern Textile Industry, 1800-1920" (PhD diss., University of South Carolina, 1977), 1-12.

57. Rosner and Markowitz, *Dying for Work*, 37; Trotter, *Coal, Class, and Color*, 88-89.

58. Reich, *A Working People*, 43.

59. For reviews of this extensive scholarship, see Kelly Lytle Hernandez, Khalil Gibran Muhammad, and Heather Ann Thompson, "Introduction: Constructing the Carceral State," *Journal of American History* 102, no. 1 (June 2015): 18-24; Kali N. Gross and Cheryl D. Hicks, "Gendering the Carceral State: African American Women, History, and the Criminal Justice System," *Journal of African American History*, 100, no. 3 (Summer 2015): 357-65.

60. Meltzer, *In Their Own Words*, 143.

61. Sarah Haley, *No Mercy Here: Gender, Punishment, and the Making of Jim Crow Modernity* (Chapel Hill: The University of North Carolina Press, 2016); Talitha L. LeFlouria, *Chained in Silence: Black Women and Convict Labor in the New South* (Chapel Hill: The University of North Carolina Press, 2015); Mary Ellen Curtin, *Black Prisoners and Their World: Alabama, 1865-1900* (Charlottesville: University Press of Virginia, 2000); Reich, *A Working People*, 48-49; Zieger, *For Jobs and Freedom*, 44-51; Harris, *The Harder We Run*, 13, 20; Douglas A. Blackmon, *Slavery by Another Name: The Re-Enslavement of Black Americans from the Civil War to World War II* (New York: Anchor Books, 2008), 1-5.

62. Quoted in Meltzer, *In Their Own Words*, 143-44, 146.

63. Leslie Brown, *Upbuilding Black Durham: Gender, Class, and Black Community Development in the Jim Crow South* (Chapel Hill: The University of North Carolina Press, 2008), 141, 144-45, 149, map, 189.

64. Powers, *Black Charlestonians*, 251; Paul S. George, "Colored Town: Miami's Black Community, 1896-1930," *The Florida Historical Quarterly* 56, no. 4 (April 1978): 432-33; N. D. B. Connolly, *A World More Concrete: Real Estate and the Remaking of Jim Crow South Florida* (Chicago: University of Chicago Press, 2014), xxx.

65. Lynne B. Feldman, *A Sense of Place: Birmingham's Black Middle Class Community, 1890-1930* (Tuscaloosa: University of Alabama Press, 1999), 24, 26-28, 71.

66. Feldman, *A Sense of Place*, 9, 19, 26-27; Rabinowitz, *Race Relations in the Urban South*, 105-06; Rice, "Residential Segregation by Law, 1910-1917," 179-82, quote, 182; Hunter, *To 'Joy My Freedom*, pp. 44-50; Massey and Denton, *American Apartheid*, 20-22.

67. L. Brown, *Upbuilding Black Durham*, 141, 144-45, 149, map, 189; Hunter, *To 'Joy My Freedom*, 46-50, 141, 144-45, 149, map, 189.

68. Darlene Clark Hine, *Black Women in White: Racial Conflict and Cooperation in the Nursing Profession, 1890-1950* (Bloomington: Indiana University Press, 1989), 8;

Borchert, *Alley Life in Washington*, 183; Chris M. Asch and George D. Musgrove, *Chocolate City: A History of Race and Democracy in the Nation's Capital* (Chapel Hill: The University of North Carolina Press, 2017), 179.

69. Rabinowitz, *Race Relations in the Urban South*, 114–24.

70. Trotter, *The African American Experience*, 307.

71. Ira Berlin, *The Making of African America: The Four Great Migrations* (New York: Viking, 2010), 152–200; Isabel Wilkerson, *The Warmth of Other Suns: The Epic Story of America's Great Migration* (New York: Random House, 2010), 8–15; Peter M. Rutkoff and William Scott, *Fly Away: The Great African American Cultural Migrations* (Baltimore: John Hopkins University Press, 2010), 11–14; James N. Gregory, *The Southern Diaspora: How the Great Migrations of Black and White Southerners Transformed America* (Chapel Hill: The University of North Carolina Press, 2005), 11–41; Johnson and Campbell, *Black Migration in America*, 71–113, 132, 158. For an illuminating perspective on these neighborhoods, see Kevin Mumford, *Interzones: Black/White Sex Districts in Chicago and New York in the Early Twentieth Century* (New York: Columbia University Press, 1997), 20–21, 23. Mumford, a historian, defines the "vice districts" as "interzones," where "tolerating prostitution" and other forms of vice "served to create a new complex of racial and gendered politics" (21).

72. McBride, *From TB to AIDS*, 10–13, 15. The next four most common causes of death among African Americans were pneumonia, diseases of the "nervous system," typhoid, and malaria (McBride, 11).

73. Washington, *Medical Apartheid*, 154; Trotter, *The African American Experience*, quote, 325–26.

74. Washington, *Medical Apartheid*, 155–56; Keith Wailoo, *Drawing Blood: Technology and Disease Identity in Twentieth-Century America* (Baltimore: Johns Hopkins University Press, 1997), 1–16.

75. McBride, *Caring for Equality*, 35.

76. McBride, 56–57.

77. The following narrative is based on Long, *Doctoring Freedom*, 114–31.

78. Long, *Doctoring Freedom*, quote, 114.

79. Long, 118.

80. Long, 126.

81. Long, 127.

82. Long, 120.

83. Long, 124.

84. Long, 129–30.

85. McBride, *Caring for Equality*, 18–19.

86. Bethel, *Promiseland*, 51.

87. Theda Skocpol, Ariane Liazos, and Marshall Ganz, *What a Mighty Power We Can Be: African American Fraternal Groups and the Struggle for Racial Equality* (Princeton, NJ: Princeton University Press, 2006), 35–37.

88. McBride, *From TB to AIDS*, 25.

89. Smith, *Sick and Tired of Being Sick and Tired*, 17–18.

90. Hine, *Black Women in White*, 19–20; McBride, *From TB to AIDS*, 26; Byrd and Clayton, *An American Health Dilemma*, 368.

91. McBride, *From TB to AIDS*, 26, quote, 28–29.

92. Long, *Doctoring Freedom*, 93–94.

93. Long, *Doctoring Freedom*, 93–94; McBride, *Caring for Equality*, 20–21.

94. Gamble, *Making Place for Ourselves*, 13; Byrd and Clayton, *An American Health Dilemma*, 326, 355, 395; McBride, *From TB to AIDS*, 25; McBride, *Caring for Equality*, 21.

95. Byrd and Clayton, *An American Health Dilemma*, 398–99.

96. Hine, *Black Women in White*, 8–9, 11–12, 24, 26–27; Gamble, *Making Place for Ourselves*, 7–8, 11; Byrd and Clayton, *An American Health Dilemma*, 102–3, 398.

97. Gamble, *Making Place for Ourselves*, 15–17; Hine, *Black Women in White*, 12, 15, 18.

98. Hine, *Black Women in White*, 34–35; Gamble, *Making Place for Ourselves*, 22.

99. L. Brown, *Upbuilding Black Durham*, 155–56, 159–60; Hine, *Black Women in White*, 8–9, 11.

100. Hine, *Black Women in White*, 9, 16–18.

101. Byrd and Clayton, *An American Health Dilemma*, 394–95.

102. Byrd and Clayton, *An American Health Dilemma*, 400–402; McBride, *Caring for Equality*, 28–29; Long, *Doctoring Freedom*, 167–77.

103. Gamble, *Making Place for Ourselves*, 10–11, 35–48; Long, *Doctoring Freedom*, 167–72; McBride, *Caring for Equality*, 39–40.

104. McBride, *From TB to AIDS*, 22–23.

105. E. Richard Brown, *Rockefeller Medicine Men: Medicine and Capitalism in America* (Berkeley: University of California Press, 1980), 148–49.

106. Starr, *The Social Transformation of American Medicine*, 124.

107. Long, *Doctoring Freedom*, 158.

108. Long, 160.

109. E. R. Brown, *Rockefeller Medicine Men*, 1–12.

Chapter Three

1. Leah Platt Boustan, *Competition in the Promised Land: Black Migrants in Northern Cities and Labor Markets* (Princeton, NJ: Princeton University Press, 2017); James N. Gregory, *The Southern Diaspora: How the Great Migrations of Black and White Southerners Transformed America* (Chapel Hill: The University of North Carolina Press, 2005); Carol Marks, *Farewell—We're Good and Gone: The Great Black Migration* (Bloomington: Indiana University Press, 1989); Isabel Wilkerson, *The Warmth of Other Suns: The Epic Story of America's Great Migration* (New York: Random House, 2010); Ira Berlin, *The Making of African America: The Four Great Migrations* (New York: Viking, 2010).

2. Allan H. Spear, *Black Chicago: The Making of a Negro Ghetto, 1890-1920* (Chicago: University of Chicago Press, 1967), quotes, 133–34.

3. All quotes appear in Joe William Trotter Jr., *The African American Experience* (Boston: Houghton Mifflin Company, 2001), 384–85.

4. Earl Lewis, *In Their Own Interests: Race, Class, and Power in Twentieth-Century Norfolk, Virginia* (Berkeley: University of California Press, 1991), 29–31; Earl Lewis, "Expectations, Economic Opportunities, and Life in the Industrial Age: Black Migration to Norfolk, Virginia, 1910-1945," in *The Great Migration in Historical Perspective: New*

Dimensions of Race, Class, and Gender, ed. Joe William Trotter Jr. (Bloomington: Indiana University Press, 1991), 22; Quintard Taylor, *In Search of the Racial Frontier: African Americans in the American West, 1528-1990* (New York: W. W. Norton, 1998), 254-55, 315; Josh Sides, *L.A. City Limits: African American Los Angeles from the Great Depression to the Present* (Berkeley: University of California Press, 2003), 15.

5. Otis Trotter, *Keeping Heart: A Memoir of Family Struggle, Race, and Medicine* (Athens: Ohio University Press, 2015), 67.

6. Darlene Clark Hine, "Black Migration in the Urban Mid-West: The Gender Dimension, 1915-1945," in *The Great Migration in Historical Perspective,* 138-39.

7. David McBride, *From TB to AIDS: Epidemics among Urban Blacks since 1900* (Albany: State University of New York Press, 1991), 38, 46-47; David Rosner and Gerald Markowitz, eds., *Dying for Work: Workers' Safety and Health in Twentieth-Century America* (Bloomington: Indiana University Press, 1989), 85.

8. W. Michael Byrd and Linda Clayton, *An American Health Dilemma: A Medical History African Americans and the Problem of Race, 1900-2000* (New York: Routledge, 2002), 154-58, 228; McBride, *From TB to AIDS,* 88, 47.

9. Samuel Kelton Roberts Jr., *Infectious Fear: Politics, Disease, and the Health Effects of Segregation* (Chapel Hill: The University of North Carolina Press, 2009). 63-64.

10. See Vanessa Northington Gamble, ed., *Germs Have No Color Line: Blacks and American Medicine, 1900-1940* (New York: Garland Publishing, 1989); Stuart Galishoff, "Germs Know No Color Line: Black Health and Public Policy in Atlanta, 1900-1918," *Journal of the History of Medicine and Allied Sciences* 40 (1985); McBride, *From TB to AIDS,* quote, 53-54; and Tera W. Hunter, *To 'Joy My Freedom: Southern Black Women's Lives and Labors after the Civil War* (Cambridge, MA: Harvard University Press, 1997), chap. 9, "Tuberculosis as the 'Negro Servants' Disease."

11. Roberts, *Infectious Fear,* 63-64; J. A. Tobey, "The Death Rates Among American Negroes," *Current History* 25, no. 2 (November 1926): 217-19; McBride, *From TB to AIDS,* 10, 53-54, 60-62, 70, 72.

12. Roberts, *Infectious Fear,* 31-32; Louis I. Dublin, "The Problem of Negro Health as Revealed by Vital Statistics," *Journal of Negro Education* 6 (1937): 268-75.

13. Dublin, "The Problem of Negro Health," 268-75; McBride, *From TB to AIDS,* 52-53.

14. McBride, *From TB to AIDS,* 71.

15. Bleecker Marquette, "Helping the Negro Solve His Problem," *The Nation's Health* 9, no. 1 (January 1927): 19-27; McBride, *From TB to AIDS,* 71-72.

16. Byrd and Clayton, *An American Health Dilemma,* 182-83; Ezelle Sanford, *Segregated Medicine: How Racial Politics Shaped American Healthcare* (book in progress, in author's possession); McBride, *From TB to AIDS,* 74.

17. Vanessa Northington Gamble, *Making Place for Ourselves: The Black Hospital Movement, 1920-1945* (New York: Oxford University Press, 1995), 105-9; Darlene Clark Hine, *Black Women in White: Racial Conflict and Cooperation in the Nursing Profession, 1890-1950* (Bloomington: Indiana University Press, 1989), 8, 10, 27, 31-34; Susan L. Smith, *Sick and Tired of Being Sick and Tired: Black Women's Health Activism in America, 1890-1950* (Philadelphia: University of Pennsylvania Press, 1995), 63-68; McBride, *From TB to AIDS,* 76, 78-79.

18. David McBride, *Caring for Equality: A History of African American Health and Healthcare* (Lanham, MD: Rowman and Littlefield, 2018), 45, 51.

19. Roberts, *Infectious Fear*, 65.

20. Edward H. Beardsley, *A History of Neglect: Health Care for Blacks and Mill Workers in the Twentieth-Century South* (Knoxville: University of Tennessee Press, 1987), 156; Steven A. Reich, *A Working People: A History of African American Workers Since Emancipation* (Lanham, MD: Rowman and Littlefield, 2013), 91; McBride, *Caring for Equality*, 60–61; Byrd and Clayton, *An American Health Dilemma*, 251.

21. Richard Walter Thomas, *Life for Us Is What We Make It: Building Black Community in Detroit, 1915-1945* (Bloomington: Indiana University Press, 1992), 28–30, 49–53, 107; August Meier and Elliot Rudwick, *Black Detroit and the Rise of the UAW* (New York: Oxford University Press, 1979), 9–16; David M. Lewis-Colman, *Race against Liberalism: Black Workers and the UAW in Detroit* (Urbana: University of Illinois Press, 2008), 5–9.

22. Thomas, *Life for Us Is What We Make It*, 28–30, 49–53, 107; Meier and Rudwick, *Black Detroit and the Rise of the UAW*; Lewis-Colman, *Race against Liberalism*, 5–9, 107.

23. Joe William Trotter Jr., *Coal, Class, and Color: Blacks in Southern West Virginia, 1915-32* (Urbana: University of Illinois Press, 1990), 106.

24. Rick Halpern, *Down on the Killing Floor: Black and White Workers in Chicago's Packinghouses, 1904-1954* (Urbana: University of Chicago Press, 1997), 179; Rick Halpern and Roger Horowitz, *Meatpackers: An Oral History of Black Packinghouse Workers and Their Struggle for Racial and Economic Equality* (New York: Twayne Publishers, 1996), 6, 33–34, 52; Allan H. Spear, *Black Chicago: The Making of a Negro Ghetto, 1890-1920* (Chicago: University of Chicago Press, 1967), 158; Roger Horowitz, "Negro and White, United and Fight!": A Social History Industrial Unionism in Meatpacking, 1930-90* (Urbana: University of Illinois Press, 1997), 23–24; Walter A. Fogel, *The Negro in the Meat Industry*, Report No. 12 (Philadelphia: University of Pennsylvania Wharton School of Finance and Commerce, 1970), 44–54.

25. Halpern and Horowitz, *Meatpackers*, 33–34.

26. Halpern and Horowitz, 33–34.

27. Thomas, *Life for Us Is What We Make It*, 106–7; Peter Gottlieb, *Making Their Own Way: Southern Blacks' Migration to Pittsburgh, 1916-30* (Urbana: University of Illinois Press, 1987), 119–20.

28. Dennis Dickerson, *Out of the Crucible: Black Steelworkers in Western Pennsylvania, 1875-1980* (Albany: State University of New York Press, 1986), 49–53; Gottlieb, *Making Their Own Way*, 96–102, 119, 124–25; Reich, *A Working People*, 67–69, quote, 71–72.

29. Rosner and Markowitz, *Dying for Work*, 70.

30. Trotter, *Coal, Class, and Color*, quote, 106; Rosner and Markowitz, *Dying for Work*, 4.

31. David Rosner and Gerald Markowitz, *Deadly Dust: Silicosis and the On-Going Struggle to Protect Workers' Health*, new and expanded edition (Ann Arbor: University of Michigan Press, 2006), 49, 70–71. ; For additional evidence on this issue, see Rosner and Markowitz, *Dying for Work*, 70–74, 96–98.

32. Jacqueline Jones, *Labor of Love, Labor of Sorrow: Black Women, Work, and the Family from Slavery to the Present* (New York: Basic Books, 1985), 167–68; Kimberley

Phillips, *Alabama North: African-American Migrants, Community, and Working Class Activism, 1915-45* (Urbana: University of Illinois Press, 1999), 72; Cheryl D. Hicks, *Talk with You Like a Woman: African American Women, Justice, and Reform in New York, 1890-1935* (Chapel Hill: The University of North Carolina Press, 2010), 39.

33. Lewis, *In Their Own Interests*, 35-37; Bernadette Pruitt, *The Other Great Migration: The Movement of Rural African Americans to Houston, 1900-1941* (College Station: Texas A&M University Press, 2013), 216; Michael Honey, *Southern Labor and Black Civil Rights: Organizing Memphis Workers, 1929-1955* (Urbana: University of Illinois Press, 1993), 35-38.

34. Leslie Brown, *Upbuilding Black Durham: Gender, Class, and Black Community Development in the Jim Crow South* (Chapel Hill: The University of North Carolina Press, 2008), 228.

35. Brown, *Upbuilding Black Durham*, 227-28.

36. Thomas, *Life for Us Is What We Make It*, 106-7.

37. Theodore Kornwiebel Jr., *Railroads in the African American Experience: A Photo Journey* (Baltimore: Johns Hopkins University Press, 2010), quote, 115-16; Jack Santino, *Miles of Smiles, Years of Struggle: Stories of Black Pullman Porters* (Urbana: University of Illinois Press, 1989), 19-21; Eric Arnesen, *Brotherhoods of Color: Black Railroad Workers and the Struggle for Equality* (Cambridge, MA: Harvard University Press, 2001), 87-88.

38. Joe William Trotter Jr., *From a Raw Deal to a New Deal?: African Americans, 1929-1945* (New York: Oxford University Press, 1996), 25-26; Quintard Taylor, *The Forging of a Black Community: Seattle's Central District from 1870 through the Civil Rights Era* (Seattle: University of Washington Press, 1994), 63.

39. Trotter, *Coal, Class, and Color*, 94.

40. Trotter, *Coal, Class, and Color*, 94.

41. Trotter, *Coal, Class, and Color*, 94.

42. Susan M. Reverby, *Examining Tuskegee: The Infamous Syphilis Study and Its Legacy* (Chapel Hill: The University of North Carolina Press, 2009), 1-10, quote, 5; Susan M. Reverby, ed., *Tuskegee's Truths: Rethinking the Tuskegee Syphilis Study* (Chapel Hill: The University of North Carolina Press, 2009), 1-11; James H. Jones, *Bad Blood: The Tuskegee Syphilis Experiment: A Tragedy of Race and Medicine* (New York: The Free Press, 1981), 1-15; Harriet A. Washington, *Medical Apartheid: The Dark History of Medical Experimentation on Black Americans from Colonial Times to the Present* (New York: Doubleday, 2006), 157-85; Byrd and Clayton, *An American Health Dilemma*, 286-90.

43. Reverby, *Tuskegee's Truths*, 1-2.

44. Reverby, 2.

45. Reverby, 2, 15, 195.

46. Jones, *Bad Blood*, 7.

47. Reverby, *Tuskegee's Truths*, 195.

48. Reverby, 195.

49. Reverby, *Examining Tuskegee*, 68.

50. Reverby, 61.

51. Reverby, 2, 282.

52. Reverby, quote, 3.

53. Reverby, *Examining Tuskegee*, 66.

54. Johanna Schoen, *Choice and Coercion: Birth Control, Sterilization, and Abortion in Public Health and Welfare* (Chapel Hill: The University of North Carolina Press, 2005), 108–9.

55. Gregory Michael Dorr, "Protection or Control?: Women's Health, Sterilization Abuse, and *Relf v. Weinberger*," in *A Century of Eugenics in America: From the Indiana Experiment to the Human Genome Era*, ed. Paul A. Lombardo (Bloomington: Indiana University Press, 2011), 161.

56. Washington, *Medical Apartheid*, 189–90; Byrd and Clayton, *An American Health Dilemma*, 285–86.

57. Byllye Avery and Susan Reverby, interview, "Ask a Feminist: Byllye Avery Discusses the Past and Future of Reproductive Justice with Susan Reverby," *Signs*, the Feminist Public Intellectuals Project, University of Chicago, 2019; Loretta Ross, interview with Byllye Y. Avery, "Voices of Feminism Oral History Project," Sophia Smith Collection, Smith College, 2006.

58. James Wolfinger, *Philadelphia Divided: Race and Politics in the City of Brotherly Love* (Chapel Hill: The University of North Carolina Press, 2007), 53, 57–58; Marcus A. Hunter, *Black Citymakers: How the Philadelphia Negro Changed Urban America* (New York: Oxford University Press, 2013), 69–71.

59. M. A. Hunter, *Black Citymakers*, 69; Wolfinger, *Philadelphia Divided*, 81, 87, 89.

60. Robert Gioielli, *Environmental Activism and the Urban Crisis: Baltimore, St. Louis, and Chicago* (Philadelphia: Temple University Press, 2014), 49; Rosner and Markowitz, *Dying for Work*, 141.

61. McBride, *From TB to AIDS*, 32, 51.

62. T. W. Hunter, *To 'Joy My Freedom*, chap. 4, "Tuberculosis as the 'Negro Servants' Disease"; Beardsley, *A History of Neglect*, 13–26; McBride, *From TB to AIDS*, 32, 51.

63. McBride, *From TB to AIDS*, 125–29.

64. For a perspective on the discriminatory treatment of Black mental health patients nationwide, see Kylie Smith, " in the Wake: Racism and the Asylum South," *Southern Spaces*, April 9, 2021; Kylie Smith, *Jim Crow in the Asylum: Psychiatry and Civil Rights in the American South* (Chapel Hill: The University of North Carolina Press, forthcoming); Martin Sommers, *Madness in the City of Magnificent Intentions: A History of Race and Mental Illness in the Nation's Capital* (New York: Oxford University Press, 2019); and Jay Garcia, *Psychology Comes to Harlem: Rethinking the Race Question in Twentieth-Century America* (Baltimore: Johns Hopkins University Press, 2012).

65. Mab Segrest, *Administrations of Lunacy: Racism and the Haunting of American Psychiatry at the Milledgeville Asylum* (New York: The New Press, 2020), 303–4.

66. Segrest, 237–38, 269.

67. Richard Rothstein, *The Color of Law: A Forgotten History of How Our Government Segregated America* (New York: Liveright Publishing/W. W. Norton, 2017), ix; Kevin McGruder, *Race and Real Estate: Conflict and Cooperation in Harlem, 1890–1920* (New York: Columbia University Press, 2015), 94, 231–32, n52; Gilbert Osofsky, *Harlem: The Making of a Ghetto, Negro New York, 1890-1930*, 2nd ed. (Chicago: Ivan R. Dee Publisher, 1996), 135–41; Allan Spear, *Black Chicago: The Making of a Negro Ghetto, 1890-1920* (Chicago: University of Chicago Press, 1967), 23; Christopher R. Reed, *The Depression*

Comes to the South Side: Protest and Politics in the Black Metropolis, 1930–1933 (Bloomington: Indiana University Press, 2011), 62.

68. Gottlieb, *Making Their Own Way*, 69–71; Robert Gregg, *Sparks from the Anvil of Oppression: Philadelphia's African Methodists and Southern Migrants, 1880–1940* (Philadelphia: Temple University Press, 1998), quote, from Carter G. Woodson, *A Century of Negro Migration* (New York: Russell and Russell, 1918), 29; Victoria Wolcott, *Remaking Respectability: African American Women in Interwar Detroit* (Chapel Hill: The University of North Carolina Press, 2001), 111; Gretchen Lemke-Santangelo, *Abiding Courage: African American Migrant Women and the East Bay Community* (Chapel Hill: The University of North Carolina Press, 1996), 81; Shirley Ann Wilson Moore, *To Place Our Deeds: The African American Community in Richmond, California, 1910–1963* (Berkeley: University of California Press, 2000), 23; Laurie B. Green, *Battling the Plantation Mentality: Memphis and the Black Freedom Struggle* (Chapel Hill: The University of North Carolina Press, 2007), 17–18.

69. McBride, *From TB to AIDS*, 37.

70. McBride, 65–66. Also see Roberts, *Infectious Fear*, 65–66.

71. Lewis, *In Their Own Interests*, 80–81; Thomas, *Life for Us Is What We Make It*, 104–5; Cheryl Lynn Greenberg, *Or Does It Explode?: Black Harlem in the Great Depression* (New York: Oxford University Press, 1991), 31–32, 186–87, 192; M. A. Hunter, *Black Citymakers*, 80–81; Dickerson, *Out of the Crucible*, 59; McBride, *From TB to AIDS*, 104.

72. Paul Starr, *The Social Transformation of American Medicine: The Rise of a Sovereign Profession and the Making of a Vast Industry* (New York: Basic Books, 1982), 124; Byrd and Clayton, *An American Health Dilemma*, 97. According to Byrd and Clayton, Abraham Flexner "proved to be [a] strict, if sometimes impulsive, critic. Virtually all agreed that although passionate, he was basically objective" (95).

73. McBride, *From TB to AIDS*, 120–21.

74. Quoted in Byrd and Clayton, *An American Health Dilemma*, 250, 264.

75. Smith, *Sick and Tired of Being Sick and Tired*, 43–57; Phoebe Ann Pollitt, "From National Negro Health Week to National Public Health Week," *Journal of Community Health* 21, no. 6 (December 1996): 401–7; Tiffany Walker, "Recovering Black History: 'National Negro Health Week,' 1915 to 1951," National Archives, Black Women and Civil Rights, March 26, 2016.

76. Gamble, *Making Place for Ourselves*, 131–50, xi–xviii, 3–19; Washington, *Medical Apartheid*, 326; Hine, *Black Women in White*, 89–90; Alondra Nelson, *Body and Soul: The Black Panther Party and the Fight against Medical Discrimination* (Minneapolis: University of Minnesota Press, 2011), 30–33.

77. Nelson, *Body and Soul*, 31–32.

78. McBride, *From TB to AIDS*, 120–21.

79. Starr, *The Social Transformation of American Medicine*, 280–81; Byrd and Clayton, *An American Health Dilemma*, 236–37; McBride, *Caring for Equality*, 76; McBride, *From TB to AIDS*, 141–44.

80. McBride, *From TB to AIDS*, 141–44.

81. Byrd and Clayton, *An American Health Dilemma*, 272.

82. McBride, *From TB to AIDS*, 141–44; Byrd and Clayton, *An American Health Dilemma*, 272.

83. Nelson, *Body and Soul*, 34–35; McBride, *From TB to AIDS*, 154–55; Byrd and Clayton, *An American Health Dilemma*, 202.

84. John Dittmer, *The Good Doctors: The Medical Committee for Human Rights and the Struggle for Social Justice in Health Care* (New York: Bloomsbury, 2009), 61, 264.

85. Dittmer, 202–3, 216; Karen Kruse Thomas, *Deluxe Jim Crow: Civil Rights and American Health Policy, 1935–1954* (Athens: University of Georgia Press, 2011), 27–29; Adam Biggs, "Desegregating Harlem Hospital: A Centennial," New York Academy of Medicine, *Book, Health, and History* (blog), August 2019; and Adams Biggs, "The Newest Negroes: Black Doctors and the Desegregation of Harlem Hospital, 1919–1935" (PhD diss., Harvard University, 2020).

86. Byrd and Clayton, *An American Health Dilemma*, 217–18, 280.

87. Gioielli, *Environmental Activism and the Urban Crisis*, 50–65, quote, 67, 81–87, 99–103.

88. Nelson, *Body and Soul*, 6, 11, 110–11; Chuck Staresinic, "Send Freedom House," *Pitt Med Magazine* (February 2004): 32–34; Phil Hallen, interview by Johanna Fernandez for CAUSE, Remembering Africanamerican Pittsburgh ("RAP"), Carnegie Mellon University, July 19, 2007; Betty Tillman, interview by Shawn Wells for CAUSE, "RAP," August 23, 2007.

89. Staresinic, "Send Freedom House"; Hallen CAUSE interview; Tillman CAUSE interview.

90. Byrd and Clayton, *An American Health Dilemma*, 203–5, 215.

91. Barbara and John Ehrenreich, *The American Health Empire: Power, Profit, and Politics* (New York: Random House, 1970), 4, cited in Byrd and Clayton, 206.

92. Byrd and Clayton, *An American Health Dilemma*, 264–71.

93. McBride, *From TB to AIDS*, 65–67, quote, 123; Byrd and Clayton, *An American Health Dilemma*, 78, 102, 130–31.

94. S. J. Holmes, "The Principal Causes of Death among Negroes: A General Comparative Statement," *Journal of Negro Education* 6 (1937): 289–302, quote, 302, reprinted in Gamble, *Germs Have No Color Line*, 150–63.

95. Byrd and Clayton, *An American Health Dilemma*, 254.

96. McBride, *Caring for Equality*, 69.

97. McBride, *From TB to AIDS*, 111, 146.

98. McBride, 146; Linda Janet Holmes, *Safe in a Midwife's Hands: Birthing Traditions from Africa to the American South* (Columbus: Mad Creek Books, Ohio State University Press 2023), 170.

99. McBride, *From TB to AIDS*, 45–46, 55–56, 69, 111–12.

100. Lewis, *In Their Own Interests*, 80.

101. This language of class is adapted from a quote by Ferdinand D. Reinhard, a Baltimore public health officer, in McBride, *From TB to AIDS*, 105.

Chapter Four

1. Gabriel Winant, *The Next Shift: The Fall of Industry and the Rise of Health Care in Rust Belt America* (Cambridge, MA: Harvard University Press, 2021), 1–24; Michael L.

Bagshaw and Robert H. Schnorbus, "The Local Labor-Market Response to a Plant Shutdown," Federal Reserve Bank of Cleveland, January 1980; Stuart Auerbach, "US Steel Set to Close Plants, End 15,000 Jobs," *Washington Post*, December 28, 1983; Steven A. Reich, *A Working People: A History of African American Workers Since Emancipation* (Lanham, MD: Rowman and Littlefield, 2013), 162.

2. Reynolds Farley, Sheldon Danziger, and Harry J. Holzer, *Detroit Divided: A Volume in the Multi-City Study of Urban Inequality* (New York: Russell Sage Foundation, 2000), 67, 69, 82; Lawrence D. Bobo, Melvin L. Oliver, James H. Johnson Jr., and Abel Valenzuela Jr., *The Prismatic Metropolis: Inequality in Los Angeles* (New York: Russell Sage Foundation, 2000), 19–20, 222; Robert H. Zieger, *For Jobs and Freedom: Race and Labor in America Since 1865* (Lexington: University Press of Kentucky, 2007), 217–18.

3. Reich, *A Working People*, 162–63.

4. Reich, *A Working People*, 162–63.

5. William J. Wilson, *When Work Disappears: The World of the New Urban Poor* (New York: Alfred A. Knopf, 1996), 15–16; Primilla Nadasen, *Household Workers Unite: The Untold Story of African American Women Who Built a Movement* (Boston: Beacon Press, 2015), 73–75, 169; William J. Wilson, *The Truly Disadvantage: The Inner City, the Underclass, and Public Policy* (Chicago: University of Chicago Press, 1987), 25–26, 172–73; Paul A. Jargowsky and Mary Jo Bane, "Ghetto Poverty in the United States, 1970–1980," in *The Urban Underclass*, ed. Christopher Jencks and Paul E. Peterson (Washington, DC: The Brookings Institution, 1991), 254–55.

6. Barbara Ransby, *Making All Black Lives Matter: Reimagining Freedom in the 21st Century* (Oakland: University of California Press, 2018), 205–6; Heather Ann Thompson, *Blood in the Water: The Attica Prison Uprising of 1971 and Its Legacy* (New York: Pantheon Books, 2016), 558–67; Elizabeth Hinton, *From the War on Poverty to the War on Crime: The Making of Mass Incarceration in America* (Cambridge, MA: Harvard University Press, 2016), 2–3; Elizabeth Hinton, *America on Fire: The Untold History of Police Violence and Black Rebellion Since the 1960s* (New York: Liveright Publishing, 2021)1–16; Michell Alexander, *The New Jim Crow: Mass Incarceration in the Age of Colorblindness* (New York: The New Press, 2010), 5–9, 52–53, 86–91.

7. Paul D. Moreno, *From Direct Action to Affirmative Action: Fair Employment Law and Policy in America, 1933-1972* (Baton Rouge: Louisiana State University Press, 1997), 188–90; Matthew Desmond, *Evicted: Poverty and Profit in the American City* (New York: Crown Publishers, 2016), 25, 208, 210; Geoffrey DeVerteuil, Heidi Sommer, Jennifer Wolch, and Lois Takahashi, "The Local Welfare State in Transition: Welfare Reform in Los Angeles," in *New York and Los Angeles: Politics, Society, and Culture, A Comparative View*, ed. David Halle (Chicago: University of Chicago Press, 2003), 269–70, 276, 282–83. Under the administration of President Ronald Reagan, the federal government cut the affirmative action enforcement powers of the Office of Federal Contract Compliance and the Equal Employment Opportunity Commission. Together, these federal, state, and local measures aimed to dismantle affirmative action programs for minorities and women and demolish the social welfare system.

8. David McBride, *Caring for Equality: A History of African American Health and Healthcare* (Lanham, MD: Rowman and Littlefield, 2018), 118–19.

9. Ira Berlin, *The Making of African America: The Four Great Migrations* (New York: Viking, 2010), 4–7, 216–25; James Campbell, *Middle Passages: African American Journeys to Africa, 1787–2005* (New York: Penguin Press, 2006), 371–73.

10. Joe William Trotter Jr., *Workers On Arrival: Black Labor in the Making of America* (Oakland: University of California Press, 2019), 166.

11. Desmond, *Evicted*, 5.

12. Andrew Wiese, *Places of Their Own: African American Suburbanization in the Twentieth Century* (Chicago: University of Chicago Press, 2004), 116–17; Douglas S. Massey and Nancy A. Denton, *American Apartheid: Segregation and the Making of the Underclass* (Cambridge, MA: Harvard University Press, 1993), 67–74; Paige Glotzer, *How the Suburbs Were Segregated: Developers and the Business of Exclusionary Housing, 1890–1960* (New York: Columbia University Press, 2020), 1–14.

13. Eric S. Brown, "The Black Professional Middle Class and the Black Community: Racialized Class Formation in Oakland and the East Bay," in *African American Urban History Since World War II*, ed. Kenneth L. Kusmer and Joe W. Trotter (Chicago: University of Chicago Press, 2009), 10–11, 263–91.

14. Keeanga-Yamahtta Taylor, *Race for Profit: How Banks and the Real Estate Industry Undermined Black Homeownership* (Chapel Hill: The University of North Carolina Press, 2019), 1–23; Jacqueline Jones, *A Dreadful Deceit: The Myth of Race from the Colonial Era to Obama's America* (New York: Basic Books, 2013), 292.

15. Jones, *A Dreadful Deceit*, 292; Sabrina Deitrick, "Cultural Change in Pittsburgh: A Demographic Analysis at City and County Scales," *Pennsylvania Geographer* 53, no. 2 (Fall–Winter 2015), 80; *ULP Report: 1999*, 8–9; Jim McKinnon, "Ex-Foes Unite Against Sanders Agreement," *Pittsburgh Post-Gazette*, May 4, 1999, accessed January 25, 2018; *ULP Report: 2000*, 8–9, 15–19; Hesalyn Hunts, Ralph Bangs, and Ken Thompson, "The Health Status of African Americans in Allegheny County: A Black Paper for the Urban League of Pittsburgh," January 2002; Trista N. Sims, "Health Problems among African American Women Age 35–64 in Allegheny County: A Black Paper for the Urban League of Pittsburgh," January 2002.

16. William J. Collins and Robert A. Margo, "The Economic Aftermath of the 1960s Riots in American Cities: Evidence from Property Values," Working Paper No. 04-w10 (Department of Economics, Vanderbilt University, Nashville, May 2004); Wiese, *Places of Their Own*, 255–92; James Borchert, *Alley Life in Washington: Family, Community, Religion, and Folklife in the City, 1850–1970* (Urbana: University of Illinois Press, 1980), 55–56; Mary Pattillo, *Black on the Block: The Politics of Race and Class in the City* (Chicago: University of Chicago Press, 2007), 1–21; Brian D. Goldstein, *The Roots of Urban Renaissance: Getrification and the Struggle over Harlem* (Cambridge, MA: Harvard University Press, 2017), 1–15.

17. Carol Stack, *Call to Home: African Americans Reclaim the Rural South* (New York: Basic Books, 1996), xi–xii, 25–26, 118; James N. Gregory, *The Southern Diaspora: How the Great Migrations of Black and White Southerners Transformed America* (Chapel Hill: The University of North Carolina Press, 2005), 322–23; Berlin, *The Making of African America*, 201–2; Isabel Wilkerson, *The Warmth of Other Suns: The Epic Story of America's Great Migration* (New York: Random House, 2010), 486–87; James S. Hirsch and Suzanne Alexander, "Reverse Exodus: Middle Class Blacks Quit Northern Cities and

Settle in the South," *Wall Street Journal*, May 22, 1990; Michelle Nickerson and Darren Dochuk, eds., *Sunbelt Rising: The Politics of Space, Place, and Region* (Philadelphia: University of Pennsylvania Press, 2011), 1–28. On the significance of age, see Wilson, *The Truly Disadvantaged*, 36–39, and for a stellar study of the reverse migration, see Sabrina Pendergrass, *The Black Reverse Migration Unfolds: Black Americans Move to the Urban South* (New York: Oxford University Press, forthcoming).

18. Paul Spickard, *Almost All Aliens: Immigration, Race, and Colonialism in American History and Identity* (New York: Routledge, 2007), quote, 385–86; Albert Camarillo, ""Blacks, Latinos, and the New Racial Frontier in American Cities of Color: California's Emerging Minority-Majority Cities," in *African American Urban History Since World War* II, 41–42; Nancy Foner, "West Indian Migration to New York: An Overview," in *Islands in the City: West Indian Migration to New York* (Berkeley: University of California Press, 2001), 3–7; Berlin, *The Making of African America*, 4–7, 216–25; Jorge Duany, *Blurred Borders: Transnational Migration Between the Hispanic Caribbean and the United States* (Chapel Hill: The University of North Carolina Press, 2011), 63–68; Campbell, *Middle Passages*, 371–73.

19. McBride, *Caring for Equality*, 118–19.

20. McBride, *Caring for Equality*, 112, 120–21.

21. W. Michael Byrd and Linda Clayton, *An American Health Dilemma: Race, Medicine, and Health Care in the United States, 1900-2000* (New York: Routledge, 2002), 556, including footnote, "H.R. 5540."

22. Linda Villarosa, *Under the Skin: The Hidden Toll of Racism on American Lives and on the Health of Our Nation* (New York: Doubleday, 2022), 18–19.

23. Villarosa, *Under the Skin*, 18–19.

24. Byrd and Clayton, *An American Health Dilemma, 1900-2000*, 555–57.

25. McBride, *Caring for Equality*, 117.

26. Ezelle Sanford, *Segregated Medicine: How Racial Politics Shaped American Healthcare* (book in progress, in author's possession); Byrd and Clayton, *An American Health Dilemma, to 1900*, 183.

27. Byrd and Clayton, *An American Health Dilemma, 1900-2000*, 414. Cf. Andrew T. Simpson, *The Medical Metropolis: Health Care and Economic Transformation in Pittsburgh and Houston* (Philadelphia: University of Pennsylvania Press, 2019), 137–48, 179–86.

28. Byrd and Clayton, *An American Health Dilemma, 1900–2000*, 555–56.

29. McBride, *Caring for Equality*, 117–18, 151.

30. Jean J. E. Bonhomme and April M. W. Young, "The Health Status of Black Men," in *Health Issues in the Black Community*, 3rd ed., ed. Ronald l. Braithwaite, Sandra E. Taylor, and Henrie M. Treadwell (San Francisco: Jossey-Bass, 2009), 80–81; McBride, *Caring for Equality*, 132–33.

31. Keith Wailoo, *Dying in the City of the Blues: Sickle Cell Anemia and the Politics of Race and Health* (Chapel Hill: The University of North Carolina Press, 2001), 9.

32. Wailoo, *Dying in the City of the Blues*, 9.

33. Keith Wailoo, *Drawing Blood: Technology and Disease Identity in Twentieth-Century America* (Baltimore: Johns Hopkins University Press, 1997), 183–85.

34. Wailoo, *Dying in the City of the Blues*, 217–18.

35. Keith Wailoo, *How Cancer Crossed the Color Line* (New York: Oxford University Press, 2011), 11.

36. Wailoo, *How Cancer Crossed the Color Line*, 11.

37. Kevin J. Mumford, *Not Straight, Not White: Black Gay Men from the March on Washington to the AIDS Crisis* (Chapel Hill: The University of North Carolina Press, 2016), 172–73; David McBride, *From TB to AIDS: Epidemics among Urban Blacks since 1900* (Albany: State University of New York Press, 1991), 163–64; Cathy J. Cohen, *The Boundaries of Blackness: AIDS and the Breakdown of Black Politics* (Chicago: University of Chicago Press, 1999), 119–48; "37th Anniversary of the First Reported Cases of AIDS in the United States," HIV.gov, June 5, 2018; Aishah Scott, "Respectability Can't Save You: The AIDS Epidemic in Black America" (PhD diss., Stony Brook University, 2019), 28, 33.

38. Cohen, *The Boundaries of Blackness*, 139–40; McBride, *From TB to AIDS*, 164–65; Scott, "Respectability Can't Save You," 28, 82; Mumford, *Not Straight, Not White*, 175.

39. Joe W. Trotter and Johanna Fernandez, "Hurricane Katrina: Urban History from the Eye of the Storm," *Journal of Urban History* 35, no. 5 (July 2009): 607–13; Chester Hartman and Gregory D. Squires, eds., *There Is No Such Thing as a Natural Disaster: Race, Class, and Hurricane Katrina* (New York: Routledge, 2006), 1–35; Jeremy I. Levitt and Matthew C. Whitaker, *Hurricane Katrina: America's Unnatural Disaster* (Lincoln: University of Nebraska Press, 2009), 1–21.

40. Kevin McQueeney, *A City Without Care: 300 Years of Racism, Health Disparities, and Health Care Activism in New Orleans* (Chapel Hill: The University of North Carolina Press, 2023), 193–94.

41. Arnold Hirsch, "(Almost) A Closer Walk with Thee: Historical Reflections on New Orleans and Hurricane Katrina," *Journal of Urban History* 35, no. 5 (July 2009); McBride, *Caring for Equality*, 149–50.

42. McBride, *Caring for Equality*, 149–50.

43. Edmund Russell, "How Does Evolutionary History Help Us Understand the Covid-19 Pandemic," *L'Indice dei Libre del Mese* (July 6, 2020), translation in author's possession, 3; Mimi Eisen, "The COVID-19 Pandemic in Historical Perspective," History Associates Incorporated, accessed spring 2021.

44. Nick Charles, "Coronavirus Rises to the Forefront for Activists in the Coronavirus Pandemic," *NBC News*, April 10, 2020.

45. Lucas Hubbard, Gwendolyn Wright, and William Darity Jr., "Introduction, Six Feet and Six Miles Apart: Structural Racism in the United States and Racially Disparate Outcomes during the COVID-19 Pandemic," in *The Pandemic Divide: How COVID Increased Inequality in America*, ed. Lucas Hubbard, Gwendolyn L. Wright, Lucas Hubbard, and William A. Darity (Durham, NC: Duke University Press, 2022), 1–28.

46. Colleen Walsh, "COVID-19 Targets Communities of Color," *Harvard Gazette: Health and Medicine*, April 11, 2020; Charles, "Coronavirus Rises to the Forefront for Activists"; Waverly Duck, Devin Rutan, and Randall Walsh, "Food Deserts and Food Oases: A Geographic Assessment of Grocery Access in American Cities" (research paper, University of Pittsburgh, Sociology Department, n.d.; Robert Manduca and Robert J. Sampson, "Childhood Exposure to Polluted Neighborhood Environments

and Intergenerational Income Mobility, Teenage Birth, and Incarceration in the USA," *Population Environment* 42 (2021): 501–23; Dorceta E. Taylor, *Toxic Communities: Environmental Racism, Industrial Pollution, and Residential Mobility* (New York: New York University Press, 2014), 140; Keisha L. Bentley-Edwards, Melissa J. Scott, and Paul A. Robbins, "How Systemic Racism and Preexisting Conditions Contributed to COVID-19 Disparities for Black Americans," in *The Pandemic Divide*, 34–35.

47. Charles, "Coronavirus Rises to the Forefront for Activists"; Walsh, "COVID-19 Targets Communities of Color."

48. Hubbard, Wright, and Darity, *The Pandemic Divide*, "Introduction," 2.

49. Donna M. Owens, "Activists Chart Course for Black America's Progress after a Year of Turmoil," *USA Today*, February 1, 2021.

50. Bentley-Edwards, Scott, and Robbins, "How Systemic Racism and Preexisting Conditions Contributed to COVID-19 Disparities for Black Americans," 35–37.

51. Hubbard, Wright, and Darity, *The Pandemic Divide*, "Introduction," 6.

52. American Psychiatric Association, "The Psychiatric Bed Crisis in the US: Understanding the Problem and Moving Toward Solutions," Section 1: Historic and Contemporary Uses of Psychiatric Beds, May 2022.

53. Mab Segrest, *Administrations of Lunacy: Racism and the Haunting of American Psychiatry at the Milledgeville Asylum* (New York: The New Press, 2020), 314–15, quote, 324, 326.

54. Jerry B. Daniel and Briggett C. Ford, "The Mental Health of African American Children, Youth, and Young Adults: What's Going on in Pittsburgh," in *The State of Black Youth in Pittsburgh: Perspectives on Young African Americans in the City of Pittsburgh and Allegheny County*, ed. Major A. Mason and Ralph L. Bangs (Pittsburgh: Urban League of Pittsburgh, 1999), 223–34; Ronald Braithwaite, Sandra E. Taylor, and Henrie M. Treadwell, eds., *Health Issues in the Black Community*, 3rd ed. (San Francisco: Jossey-Bass, 2009), especially the specialized essays on the health status of African American children, adolescents, men, and women, 35–95; Nancy Krieger, Anna Kosheleva, Pamela D. Waterman, Jarvis T. Chen, and Karestan Koenen, "Racial Discrimination, Psychological Distress, and Self-Rated Health Among US-Born and Foreign-Born Black Americans," *American Journal of Public Health* 101, no. 9 (September 2011): 1704–13; and David R. William, Yan Yu, James S. Jackson, and Norman B. Anderson, "Racial Differences in Physical and Mental Health: Socio-Economic Status, Stress and Discrimination," *Journal of Health Psychology* 2, no. 3 (1997): 335–51.

55. John Hennen, *A Union for Appalachian Healthcare Workers: The Radical Roots and Hard Fights of Local 1199* (Morgantown: West Virginia University Press, 2021), 1–2, 50; Leon Fink and Brian Greenberg, *Upheaval in the Quiet Zone: A History of Hospital Workers' Union, Local 1199* (Urbana: University of Illinois Press, 1989), 129–58.

56. Hennen, *A Union for Appalachian Healthcare Workers*, 1–2, 50; Winant, *The Next Shift*, 152–53; Fink and Greenberg, *Upheaval in the Quiet Zone*, 129–58.

57. Hennen, *A Union for Appalachian Healthcare Workers*, 1–2, 50; Winant, *The Next Shift*, 152–53; Fink and Greenberg, *Upheaval in the Quiet Zone*, 129–58.

58. Rhonda Y. Williams, *The Politics of Public Housing: Black Women's Struggles against Urban Inequality* (New York: Oxford University Press, 2004), 222–28.

59. Trotter, *Workers On Arrival*, 170–71; Brian Purnell, "Unmaking the Ghetto: Community Development and Persistent Social Inequality in Brooklyn, Los Angeles, and Philadelphia," in *The Ghetto in Global History: 1500 to the Present*, ed. Wendy Z. Goldman and Joe W. Trotter (New York: Routledge, 2017), 256–74.

60. Richard Walter Thomas, "The Black Community Building Process in Post-Urban Disorder Detroit, 1967–1997," in *African American Urban Experience: Perspectives from the Colonial Era to the Present*, ed. Joe W. Trotter, Earl Lewis, and Tera Hunter (New York: Palgrave/Macmillan, 2004), 209–40; D. G. Kelley, *Yo' Mama's Disfunktional!: Fighting the Culture Wars in Urban America* (New York: Beacon, 1997), 146–47; Thomas Sugrue, *Sweet Land of Liberty: The Forgotten Struggle for Civil Rights in the North* (New York: Random House, 2009), 525.

61. Byrd and Clayton, *An American Health* Dilemma, 557; McBride, *Caring for Equality*, 128–29.

62. Byrd and Clayton, *An American Health Dilemma*, 557; McBride, *Caring for Equality*, 128–29.

63. This and the next three paragraphs draw upon Joe William Trotter Jr., *Pittsburgh and the Urban League Movement: A Century of Social Service and Activism* (Lexington: University Press of Kentucky, 2020), 159–79.

64. Trotter, *Pittsburgh and the Urban League Movement*, 159–79.

65. Trotter, *Pittsburgh and the Urban League Movement*, 159–79.

66. Robert Gioielli, *Environmental Activism and the Urban Crisis: Baltimore, St. Louis, and Chicago* (Philadelphia: Temple University Press, 2014), 50–65, 81–87, 99–103; McBride, *Caring for Equality*, 140.

67. Marcus A. Hunter, *Black Citymakers: How the Philadelphia Negro Changed Urban America* (New York: Oxford University Press, 2013); Jeffrey Helgeson, *Crucibles of Black Empowerment: Chicago's Neighborhood Politics from the New Deal to Harold Washington* (Chicago: University of Chicago Press, 2014); Zieger, *For Jobs and Freedom*, 233; Nancy Maclean, *Freedom Is Not Enough: The Opening of the American Workplace* (New York: Russell Sage and Harvard University Press, 2006), 289–90; Jacqueline Jones, *American Work: Four Centuries of Black and White Labor* (New York: W. W. Norton, 1998), 370; David R. Colburn and Jeffrey S. Adler, *African American Mayors: Race, Politics, and the American City* (Urbana: University of Illinois Press, 2005); David O. Sears, "Black-White Conflict: A Model for the Future of Ethnic Politics in Los Angeles," in *New York and Los Angeles: Politics, Society, and Culture, A Comparative View*, ed. David Halle (Chicago: University of Chicago Press, 2003), 370–71, 375–76; Matthew Countryman, *Up South: Civil Rights and Black Power in Philadelphia* (Philadelphia: University of Pennsylvania Press, 2006), 323–25; Hunter, *Black Citymakers*, 180–89; Sugrue, *Sweet Land of Liberty*, 504–5; Roger Biles, "Mayor David Dinkins and the Politics of Race in New York City," in Colburn and Adler, *African American Mayors*, 130–52; Karen M. Kaufmann, "The Mayoral Politics of New York and Los Angeles," in Halle, ed., *New York and Los Angeles*, 324–29; Wilkerson, *The Warmth of Other Suns*, 529; Hunter, *Black Citymakers*, 187–89.

68. McBride, *Caring for Equality*, 122–23.

69. Wailoo, *Dying in the City of the Blues*, 192.

70. Wailoo, *How Cancer Crossed the Color Line*, 142–43.

71. Wailoo, *How Cancer Crossed the Color Line*, 142–43.

72. McBride, *From TB to AIDS*, 166–67; McBride, *Caring for Equality*, 136, 141.

73. McBride, *From TB to AIDS*, 166–67; McBride, *Caring for Equality*, 136, 141.

74. McBride, *From TB to AIDS*, 166–69; Cohen, *The Boundaries of Blackness*, 111–18; Scott, "Respectability Can't Save You," 83–98.

75. McBride, *From TB to AIDS*, 166–69; Cohen, *The Boundaries of Blackness*, 111–18; Scott, "Respectability Can't Save You," 83–98.

76. McQueeney, *A City Without Care*, 194. Other founding members of the clinic included Scott Crow, Sharon Johnson, and Ferris Bowles.

77. Ari Kelman, "Even Paranoids Have Enemies: Rumors of Levee Sabotage in New Orleans's Lower Ninth Ward," *Journal of Urban History* 35, no. 5 (July 2009).

78. Kelman, "Even Paranoids Have Enemies."

79. Kelman, "Even Paranoids Have Enemies."

80. Farah Jasmine Griffin, "Children of Omar: Resistance and Reliance in the Expressive Cultures of Black New Orleans," *Journal of Urban History* 35, no. 5 (July 2009).

81. Griffin, "Children of Omar."

82. Danille K. Taylor, "'Chocolate City': Personal Reflections from New Orleans, August 29, 2006," *Journal of Urban History* 35, no. 5 (July 2009).

83. Taylor, "'Chocolate City'"; McBride, *Caring for Equality*, 152.

84. Sandra Barnes, "'God Is in Control': Race. Religion, Family, and Community during the Covid-19 Pandemic," in *The Pandemic Divide*, 81–82.

85. Barnes, "'God Is in Control,'" quotes, 74–75, 79.

86. Linda Janet Holmes, *Safe in a Midwife's Hands: Birthing Traditions from Africa to the American South* (Columbus: Mad Creek Books, Ohio State University Press, 2023), ix–xii.

87. Owens, "Activists Chart Course for Black America's Progress."

88. Akilah Johnson and Sabrina Malhi, "US Life Expectancy Down for 2nd Year," *Pittsburgh Post-Gazette*, September 1, 2022.

89. Ta-Nehisi Coates, *We Were Eight Years in Power: An American Tragedy* (New York: One World Press, 2017).

90. Walda Katz-Fishman, Jerome Scott, Ralph C. Gomes, and Robert Newby, "The Politics of Race and Class in City Hall," in Jerry Lemkcke, ed., *Race, Class, and Urban Change*, Vol. 1 (Greenwich, CT: JAI Press Inc., 1989), 150–51; Kleppner, *Chicago Divided*, 145, 154; McBride, *Caring for Equality Freedom*, 152.

91. Elizabeth Day, "#BlacklivesMatter: The Birth of a New Civil Rights Movement," *The Guardian*, July 19, 2015, accessed December 28, 2017; Clarence Lang, *Black America in the Shadow of the Sixties: Notes on the Civil Rights Movement, Neoliberalism, and Politics* (Ann Arbor: University of Michigan, 2015), xv, 13, 34, 126–27, 130; quote in Bryan Tarnowski and Janell Ross, "Black Lives Matter Shifts from Protests to Policy under Trump," *Washington Post*, May 2017. Also see Brandon E. Patterson, "How the Black Lives Matter Movement Is Mobilizing Against Trump," *Mother Jones*, February 7, 2017.

92. Roger A. Mitchell Jr. and Jay D. Aronson, *Death in Custody: How America Ignores the Truth and What We Can Do about It* (Baltimore: John Hopkins University Press, 2023), 2.

Conclusion

1. David McBride, *From TB to AIDS: Epidemics among Urban Blacks since 1900* (Albany: State University of New York Press, 1991), 18–21.

2. W. E. B. Du Bois, *The Philadelphia Negro: A Social Study* (1899; repr. Philadelphia: University of Pennsylvania Press, 1996), quotes, 163.

3. Gunnar Myrdal, *An American Dilemma: The Negro Problem and Modern Democracy, Volume I* (1944; repr. New York: Pantheon Books, 1962), quote, 171–72.

4. Gerald David Jaynes and Robin M. William Jr., *A Common Destiny: Blacks and American Society* (Washington, DC: National Academy Press, 1989), 4, 21.

5. Ronald L. Braithwaite, Sandra E. Taylor, and Henrie M. Treadwell, eds., *Health Issues in the Black Community*, 3rd ed. (San Francisco: Jossey-Bass, 2009), xvii.

6. Rana A. Hogarth, *Medicalizing Blackness: Making Racial Difference in the Atlantic World, 1780-1840* (Chapel Hill: The University of North Carolina Press, 2017), 190–91.

7. Barbara J. Fields, "Origins of the New South and the Negro Question," *Journal of Southern History* 67 (2001): 811–26, quoted in Margaret Humphreys, *Intensely Human: The Health of the Black Soldier in the American Civil War* (Baltimore: Johns Hopkins University Press, 2008), 40.

8. W. Michael Byrd and Linda A. Clayton, *An American Health Dilemma: A Medical History of African Americans and the Problem of Race, Beginnings to 1900* (New York: Routledge, 2000), chaps. 3–5.

9. Jim Downs, *Sick from Freedom: African-American Illness and Suffering during the Civil War and Reconstruction* (New York: Oxford University Press, 2012).

10. Leah Platt Bouston, *Competition in the Promised Land: Black Migrants in Northern Cities and Labor Markets* (Princeton, NJ: Princeton University Press, 2017); Isabel Wilkerson, *The Warmth of Other Suns: The Epic Story of America's Great Migration* (New York: Random House, 2010); Ira Berlin, *The Making of African America: The Four Great Migrations* (New York: Viking, 2010); Steven A. Reich, *A Working People: A History of African American Workers since Emancipation* (Lanham, MD: Rowman and Littlefield, 2013); James R. Grossman, *Land of Hope: Chicago, Black Southerners, and the Great Migration* (Chicago: University of Chicago Press, 1989).

11. Harriet A. Washington, *Medical Apartheid: The Dark History of Medical Experimentation on Black Americans from Colonial Times to the Present* (New York: Doubleday, 2006); James H. Jones, *Bad Blood: The Tuskegee Syphilis Experiment: A Tragedy of Race and Medicine* (New York: The Free Press, 1981).

12. Gwendolyn L. Wright, Lucas Hubbard, and William A. Darity Jr., *The Pandemic Divide: How Covid Increased Inequality in America* (Durham, NC: Duke University Press, 2022), 1–26.

13. Joe W. Trotter and Jared N. Day, *Race and Renaissance: African Americans in Pittsburgh since World War II* (Pittsburgh: University of Pittsburgh Press, 2010), 146.

14. For this quote, and others in the remainder of this conclusion, see Gabriel Winant, *The Next Shift: The Fall of Industry and the Rise of Health Care in Rust Belt America* (Cambridge, MA: Harvard University Press, 2021), 256, 262–64.

15. Sharla Fett, *Working Cures: Healing, Health, and Power on Southern Slave Plantations* (Chapel Hill: The University of North Carolina Press, 2002); Gretchen Long,

Doctoring Freedom: The Politics of African American Medical Care in Slavery and Freedom (Chapel Hill: The University of North Carolina Press, 2012).

16. Theda Skocpol, Ariane Liazos, and Marshall Ganz, *What a Mighty Power We Can Be: African American Fraternal Groups and the Struggle for Racial Equality* (Princeton, NJ: Princeton University Press, 2006); Susan L. Smith, *Sick and Tired of Being Sick and Tired: Black Women's Health Activism in America, 1890–1950* (Philadelphia: University of Pennsylvania Press, 1995).

17. Alondra Nelson, *Body and Soul: The Black Panther Party and the Fight against Medical Discrimination* (Minneapolis: University of Minnesota Press, 2011).

18. Barbara Ransby, *Making All Black Lives Matter: Reimagining Freedom in the 21st Century* (Oakland: University of California Press, 2018).

Selected Bibliography

Adams, Catherine, and Elizabeth H. Pleck. *Love of Freedom: Black Women in Colonial and Revolutionary New England.* New York: Oxford University Press, 2010.

Alexander, Michelle. *The New Jim Crow: Mass Incarceration in the Age of Colorblindness.* New York: The Free Press, 2010.

Asch, Chris M., and George D. Musgrove. *Chocolate City: A History of Race and Democracy in the Nation's Capital.* Chapel Hill: The University of North Carolina Press, 2017.

Beardsley, Edward H. *A History of Neglect: Health Care for Blacks and Mill Workers in the Twentieth-Century South.* Knoxville: University of Tennessee Press, 1987.

Benjamin, Georges C. "Foreword." In *Health Issues in the Black Community*, 3rd ed., edited by Ronald L. Braithwaite, Sandra E. Taylor, and Henrie M. Treadwell. San Francisco: Jossey-Bass, 2009.

Berlin, Ira. *The Making of African America: The Four Great Migrations.* New York: Viking, 2010.

———. *Many Thousands Gone: The First Two Centuries of Slavery in North America.* Cambridge: Belknap Press, 1998.

———. *Slaves Without Masters: The Free Negro in the Antebellum South.* New York: Oxford University Press, 1974.

Berlin, Ira, and Philip D. Morgan. *Cultivation and Culture: Labor and the Shaping of Slave Life in the Americas.* Charlottesville: University of Virginia Press, 1993.

Berry, Daina Ramey. *The Price for Their Pound of Flesh: The Value of the Enslaved from Womb to Grave, in the Building of the Nation.* Boston: Beacon Press, 2017.

Blassingame, John. *Black New Orleans, 1865–1880.* Chicago: University of Chicago Press, 1973.

Bobo, Lawrence D., Melvin L. Oliver, James H. Johnson Jr., and Abel Valenzuela Jr. *The Prismatic Metropolis: Inequality in Los Angeles.* New York: Russell Sage Foundation, 2000.

Boustan, Leah Platt. *Competition in the Promised Land: Black Migrants in Northern Cities and Labor Markets.* Princeton, NJ: Princeton University Press, 2017.

Braithwaite, Ronald L., Sandra E. Taylor, and Henrie M. Treadwell, eds. *Health Issues in the Black Community*, 3rd ed. San Francisco: Jossey-Bass, 2009.

Brown, Leslie. *Upbuilding Black Durham: Gender, Class, and Black Community Development in the Jim Crow South.* Chapel Hill: The University of North Carolina Press, 2008.

Byrd, Alexander X. *Captives and Voyagers: Black Migrants Across the Eighteenth-Century British Atlantic World.* Baton Rouge: Louisiana State University Press, 2008.

Byrd, W. Michael, and Linda Clayton. *An American Health Dilemma: A Medical History of African Americans and the Problem of Race, Beginnings to 1900.* New York: Routledge, 2000.

————. *An American Health Dilemma: Race, Medicine, and Health Care in the United States 1900–2000*. New York: Routledge, 2002.

Carter, Chelsey, and Ezelle Sanford III. "The Myth of Black Immunity: Racialized Disease During the COVID-19 Pandemic." African American Intellectual History Society (AAIHS). Blog post, April 3, 2020.

Coates, Ta-Nehisi. *We Were Eight Years in Power: An American Tragedy*. New York: One World Press, 2017.

Cobb, James C. *The Most Southern Place on Earth: The Mississippi Delta and the Roots of Regional Identity*. New York: Oxford University Press, 1992.

Cohen, Cathy J. *The Boundaries of Blackness: AIDS and the Breakdown of Black Politics*. Chicago: University of Chicago Press, 1999.

Curry, Leonard P. *The Free Black Urban America, 1800–1850: The Shadow of the Dream*. Chicago: University of Chicago Press, 1981.

Dabel, Jane E. *A Respectable Woman: The Public Roles of African American Women in Nineteenth-Century New York*. New York: New York University Press, 2008.

Desmond, Matthew. *Evicted: Poverty and Profit in the American City*. New York: Crown Publishers, 2016.

Dittmer, John. *The Good Doctors: The Medical Committee for Human Rights and the Struggle for Social Justice in Health Care*. New York: Bloomsbury, 2009.

Downs, Jim. *Sick from Freedom: African-American Illness and Suffering during the Civil War and Reconstruction*. New York: Oxford University Press, 2012.

Drake, St. Clair, and Horace R. Cayton. *Black Metropolis: A Study of Negro Life in a Northern City*. Chicago: University of Chicago Press, 1993. Originally published 1945.

Du Bois, W. E. B. *The Philadelphia Negro: A Social Study*. Philadelphia: University of Pennsylvania Press, 1996. Originally published 1899.

Farley, Reynolds, Sheldon Danziger, and Harry J. Holzer. *Detroit Divided: A Volume in the Multi-City Study of Urban Inequality*. New York: Russell Sage Foundation, 2000.

Fett, Sharla. *Working Cures: Healing, Health, and Power on Southern Slave Plantations*. Chapel Hill: The University of North Carolina Press, 2002.

Fink, Leon, and Brian Greenberg. *Upheaval in the Quiet Zone: A History of Hospital Workers' Union, Local 1199*. Urbana: University of Illinois Press, 1989.

Foner, Philip S. *Organized Labor and the Black Worker, 1619–1973*. New York: Praeger Publishers, 1974.

Galishoff, Stuart. "Germs Know No Color Line: Black Health and Public Policy in Atlanta, 1900–1918." *Journal of the History of Medicine and Allied Sciences* 40 (1985).

Gamble, Vanessa Northington. *Making Place for Ourselves: The Black Hospital Movement, 1920–1945*. New York: Oxford University Press, 1995.

————, ed. *Germs Have No Color Line: Blacks and American Medicine, 1900–1940*. New York: Garland Publishing, 1989.

Gioielli, Robert. *Environmental Activism and the Urban Crisis: Baltimore, St. Louis, and Chicago*. Philadelphia: Temple University Press, 2014.

Glotzer, Paige. *How the Suburbs Were Segregated: Developers and the Business of Exclusionary Housing, 1890–1960*. New York: Columbia University Press, 2020.

Greenberg, Cheryl Lynn. *Or Does It Explode?: Black Harlem in the Great Depression.* New York: Oxford University Press, 1991.

Gregg, Robert. *Sparks from the Anvil of Oppression: Philadelphia's African Methodists and Southern Migrants, 1880–1940.* Philadelphia: Temple University Press, 1998.

Gregory, James N. *The Southern Diaspora: How the Great Migrations of Black and White Southerners Transformed America.* Chapel Hill: The University of North Carolina Press, 2005.

Grossman, James. *Land of Hope: Chicago, Black Southerners, and the Great Migration.* Chicago: University of Chicago Press, 1989.

Hahn, Steven. *A Nation Under Our Feet: Black Political Struggles in the Rural South from Slavery to the Great Migration.* Cambridge, MA: Harvard University Press, 2003.

Halpern, Rick. *Down on the Killing Floor: Black and White Workers in Chicago's Packinghouses, 1904–1954.* Urbana: University of Illinois Press, 1997.

Halpern, Rick, and Roger Horowitz. *Meatpackers: An Oral History of Black Packinghouse Workers and Their Struggle for Racial and Economic Equality.* New York: Twayne Publishers, 1996.

Hammonds, Evelyn M., and Rebecca M. Herzig, eds. *The Nature of Difference: Sciences of Race in the United States from Jefferson to Genomics.* Cambridge, MA: MIT Press, 2008.

Hennen, John. *A Union for Appalachian Healthcare Workers: The Radical Roots and Hard Fights of Local 1199.* Morgantown: West Virginia University Press, 2021.

Hine, Darlene Clark. *Black Women in White: Racial Conflict and Cooperation in the Nursing Profession, 1890–1950.* Bloomington: Indiana University Press, 1989.

Hinton, Elizabeth. *America on Fire: The Untold History of Police Violence and Black Rebellion Since the 1960s.* New York: Liveright Publishing, 2021.

———. *From the War on Poverty to the War on Crime: The Making of Mass Incarceration in America.* Cambridge, MA: Harvard University Press, 2016.

Hogarth, Rana A. *Medicalizing Blackness: Making Racial Difference in the Atlantic World, 1780–1840.* Chapel Hill: The University of North Carolina Press, 2017.

Holmes, Linda Janet. *Safe in a Midwife's Hands: Birthing Traditions from Africa to the American South.* Columbus: Mad Creek Books, Ohio State University Press, 2023.

Honey, Michael. *Southern Labor and Black Civil Rights: Organizing Memphis Workers, 1929–1955.* Urbana: University of Illinois Press, 1993.

Horton, James Oliver, and Lois E. Horton. *In Hope of Liberty: Culture, Community, and Protest among Northern Free Blacks, 1700–1860.* New York: Oxford University Press, 1997.

Hubbard, Lucas, Gwendolyn Wright, and William Darity, Jr., ed. *The Pandemic Divide: How COVID Increased Inequality in America.* Durham: Duke University Press, 2022.

Humphreys, Margaret. *Intensely Human: The Health of the Black Soldier in the American Civil War.* Baltimore: Johns Hopkins University Press, 2008.

Hunter, Tera W. *To 'Joy My Freedom: Southern Black Women's Lives and Labors after the Civil War.* Cambridge, MA: Harvard University Press, 1997.

Jaynes, Gerald David, and Robin M. William Jr. *A Common Destiny: Blacks and American Society.* Washington, DC: National Academy Press, 1989.

Johnson, Walter. *River of Dark Dreams: Slavery and Empire in the Cotton Kingdom*. Cambridge, MA: The Belknap Press of Harvard University, 2013.

Johnson, Whittington B. *Black Savannah, 1788-1864*. Fayetteville: University of Arkansas Press, 1996.

Jones, Jacqueline. *American Work: Four Centuries of Black and White Labor*. New York: W. W. Norton, 1998.

Jones, James H. *Bad Blood: The Tuskegee Syphilis Experiment: A Tragedy of Race and Medicine*. New York: The Free Press, 1981.

Kennedy, Cynthia M. *Braided Relations, Entwined Lives: The Women of Charleston's Urban Slave Society*. Bloomington: Indiana University Press, 2005.

Kenny, Stephen C. "The Development of Medical Museums in the Antebellum American South: Slave Bodies in Networks of Anatomical Exchange." *Bulletin of the History of Medicine* 87 (Spring 2013): 32–62.

King, Wilma. *The Essence of Liberty: Free Black Women during the Slave Era*. Columbia: University of Missouri Press, 2006.

Lang, Clarence. *Black America in the Shadow of the Sixties: Notes on the Civil Rights Movement, Neoliberalism, and Politics*. Ann Arbor: University of Michigan, 2015.

Lebsock, Suzanne. *The Free Women of Petersburg: Status and Culture in a Southern Town, 1784-1860*. New York: Norton, 1984.

Lembcke, Jerry. *Race, Class, and Urban Change*, Vol. I. Greenwich, CT: JAI Press, 1989.

Lemke-Santangelo. *Abiding Courage: African American Migrant Women and the East Bay Community*. Chapel Hill: The University of North Carolina Press, 1996.

Lewis, Earl. *In Their Own Interests: Race, Class, and Power in Twentieth-Century Norfolk, Virginia*. Berkeley: University of California Press, 1991.

Lewis, Ronald L. *Coal, Iron, and Slaves: Industrial Slavery in Maryland and Virginia, 1715-1865*. Westport, CT: Greenwood Press, 1979.

Lewis-Colman, David M. *Race against Liberalism: Black Workers and the UAW in Detroit*. Urbana: University of Illinois Press, 2008.

Lombardo, Paul A. *A Century of Eugenics in America: From the Indiana Experiment to the Human Genome Era*. Bloomington: Indiana University Press, 2011.

Long, Gretchen. *Doctoring Freedom: The Politics of African American Medical Care in Slavery and Freedom*. Chapel Hill: The University of North Carolina Press, 2012.

Marks, Carol. *Farewell — We're Good and Gone: The Great Black Migration*. Bloomington: Indiana University Press, 1989.

Massey, Douglas S., and Nancy A. Denton. *American Apartheid: Segregation and the Making of the Underclass*. Cambridge, MA: Harvard University Press, 1993.

McBride, David. *Caring for Equality: A History of African American Health and Healthcare*. Lanham, MD: Rowman and Littlefield, 2018.

———. *From TB to AIDS: Epidemics among Urban Blacks since 1900*. Albany: State University of New York Press, 1991.

McQueeney, Kevin. *A City without Care: 300 Years of Racism, Health Disparities, and Health Care Activism in New Orleans*. Chapel Hill: The University of North Carolina Press, 2023.

Meier, August, and Elliot Rudwick. *Black Detroit and the Rise of the UAW*. New York: Oxford University Press, 1979.

Moreno, Paul D. *From Direct Action to Affirmative Action: Fair Employment Law and Policy in America, 1933–1972*. Baton Rouge: Louisiana State University Press, 1997.

Morgan, Philip D. *Slave Counterpoint: Black Culture in the Eighteenth-Century Chesapeake and Lowcountry*. Chapel Hill: The University of North Carolina Press, 1998.

Mumford, Kevin J. *Not Straight, Not White: Black Gay Men from the March on Washington to the AIDS Crisis*. Chapel Hill: The University of North Carolina Press, 2016.

Myrdal, Gunnar. *An American Dilemma: The Negro Problem and Modern Democracy, Volume I*. New York: Pantheon Books, 1944. Reprinted 1962.

Nadasen, Primilla. *Household Workers Unite: The Untold Story of African American Women Who Built a Movement*. Boston: Beacon Press, 2015.

Nash, Gary. *Forging Freedom: The Formation of Philadelphia's Black Community, 1720–1840*. Cambridge, MA: Harvard University Press, 1988.

Nelson, Alondra. *Body and Soul: The Black Panther Party and the Fight against Medical Discrimination*. Minneapolis: University of Minnesota Press, 2011.

Newman, Richard S. *Freedom's Prophet: Bishop Richard Allen, the A. M. E. Church, and the Black Founding Fathers*. New York: New York University Press, 2008.

Olwell, Robert. *Masters, Slaves, and Subjects: South Carolina Low Country, 1740–1790*. Ithaca, NY: Cornell University Press, 1998.

Owens, Deirdre Cooper. *Medical Bondage: Race, Gender, and the Origins of American Gynecology*. Athens: University of Georgia Press, 2017.

Phillips, Christopher. *Freedom's Port: The African American Community of Baltimore, 1790–1860*. Urbana: University of Illinois Press, 1997.

Powers, Bernard E., Jr. *Black Charlestonians: A Social History, 1822–1885*. Fayetteville: University of Arkansas Press, 1994.

Pruitt, Bernadette. *The Other Great Migration: The Movement of Rural African Americans to Houston, 1900–1941*. College Station: Texas A&M University Press, 2013.

Ransby, Barbara. *Making All Black Lives Matter: Reimagining Freedom in the 21st Century*. Oakland: University of California Press, 2018.

Rediker, Marcus. *The Slave Ship: A Human History*. New York: Viking, 2007.

Reich, Steven A. *A Working People: A History of African American Workers Since Emancipation*. Lanham, MD: Rowman and Littlefield, 2013.

Roberts, Samuel Kelton, Jr. *Infectious Fear: Politics, Disease, and the Health Effects of Segregation*. Chapel Hill: The University of North Carolina Press, 2009.

Rockman, Seth. *Scraping By: Wage Labor, Slavery, and Survival in Early Baltimore*. Baltimore, MD: Johns Hopkins University Press, 2009.

Saville, Julie. *The Work of Reconstruction: From Slave to Wage Laborer in South Carolina, 1860–1870*. Cambridge, MA: Cambridge University Press, 1996.

Savitt, Todd L. *Medicine and Slavery: The Diseases and Health Care of Blacks in Antebellum Virginia*. Urbana: University of Illinois Press, 1978.

Schoen, Johanna. *Choice and Coercion: Birth Control, Sterilization, and Abortion in Public Health and Welfare*. Chapel Hill: The University of North Carolina Press, 2005.

Schweninger, Loren L. *Black Property Owners in the South, 1790–1915*. Urbana: University of Illinois Press, 1990.

Scott, Aishah. "Respectability Can't Save You: The AIDS Epidemic in Black America." PhD diss. Stony Brook University, 2019.

Segrest, Mab. *Administrations of Lunacy: Racism and the Haunting of American Psychiatry at the Milledgeville Asylum*. New York: The New Press, 2020.

Sides, Josh. *L.A. City Limits: African American Los Angeles from the Great Depression to the Present*. Berkeley: University of California Press, 2003.

Skocpol, Theda, Ariane Liazos, and Marshall Ganz. *What a Mighty Power We Can Be: African American Fraternal Groups and the Struggle for Racial Equality*. Princeton, NJ: Princeton University Press, 2006.

Smallwood, Stephanie E. *Saltwater Slavery: A Middle Passage from Africa to American Diaspora*. Cambridge, MA: Harvard University Press, 2007.

Smith, Susan L. *Sick and Tired of Being Sick and Tired: Black Women's Health Activism in America, 1890–1950*. Philadelphia: University of Pennsylvania Press, 1995.

Starr, Paul. *The Social Transformation of American Medicine: The Rise of a Sovereign Profession and the Making of a Vast Industry*. New York: Basic Books, 1982.

Taylor, Dorceta E. *The Environment and the People in American Cities, 1600s–1900s*. Durham, NC: Duke University Press, 2009.

Taylor, Keeanga-Yamahtta. *Race for Profit: How Banks and the Real Estate Industry Undermined Black Homeownership*. Chapel Hill: The University of North Carolina Press, 2019.

Taylor, Quintard. *In Search of the Racial Frontier: African Americans in the American West, 1528–1990*. New York: W. W. Norton, 1998.

Thomas, Richard Walter. *Life for Us Is What We Make It: Building Black Community in Detroit, 1915–1945*. Bloomington: Indiana University Press, 1992.

Thompson, Heather Ann. *Blood in the Water: The Attica Prison Uprising of 1971 and Its Legacy*. New York: Pantheon Books, 2016.

Trotter, Joe William, Jr. *The African American Experience*. Boston: Houghton Mifflin, 2001.

———. *Coal, Class, and Color: Blacks in Southern West Virginia, 1915–32*. Urbana: University of Illinois Press, 1990.

———. *Pittsburgh and the Urban League Movement: A Century of Social Service and Activism*. Lexington: University Press of Kentucky, 2020.

———. *Workers On Arrival: Black Labor in the Making of America*. Oakland: University of California Press, 2019.

Wade, Richard C. *Slavery in the Cities: The South, 1820–1860*. London: Oxford University Press, 1964.

Walker, Juliet E. K. *The History of Black Business in America: Capitalism, Race, Entrepreneurship, Vol. 1, to 1865*. 2nd ed. Chapel Hill: The University of North Carolina Press, 2009.

Washington, Harriet. *Medical Apartheid: The Dark History of Medical Experimentation on Black Americans from Colonial Times to the Present*. New York: Doubleday, 2006.

Whitman, T. Stephen. *The Price of Freedom: Slavery and Manumission in Baltimore and Early National Maryland*. Lexington: University Press of Kentucky, 1997.

Wiese, Andrew. *Places of Their Own: African American Suburbanization in the Twentieth Century*. Chicago: University of Chicago Press, 2004.

Wilkerson, Isabel. *The Warmth of Other Suns: The Epic Story of America's Great Migration*. New York: Random House, 2010.

Williams, Rhonda Y. *The Politics of Public Housing: Black Women's Struggles against Urban Inequality*. New York: Oxford University Press, 2004.

Wilson, William J. *The Truly Disadvantaged: The Inner City, the Underclass, and Public Policy*. Chicago: University of Chicago Press, 1987.

———. *When Work Disappears: The World of the New Urban Poor*. New York: Alfred A. Knopf, 1996.

Winant, Gabriel. *The Next Shift: The Fall of Industry and the Rise of Health Care in Rust Belt America*. Cambridge, MA: Harvard University Press, 2021.

Winch, Julie. *Philadelphia's Black Elite: Activism, Accommodation, and the Struggle for Autonomy, 1787-1848*. Philadelphia: Temple University Press, 1988.

Wood, Peter. *Black Majority: Negroes in Colonial South Carolina from 1670 through the Stono Rebellion*. New York: W. W. Norton, 1974.

Woodruff, Nan Elizabeth. *American Congo: The African American Freedom Struggle in the Delta*. Cambridge, MA: Harvard University Press, 2003.

Woodson, Carter G. *A Century of Negro Migration*. New York: Russell and Russell, 1918.

Zieger, Robert H. *For Jobs and Freedom: Race and Labor in America since 1865*. Lexington: University Press of Kentucky, 2007.

Index

Italic page numbers refer to illustrations.

Bacon, Alice Mabel, 76
Bacon, Charles S., 51
Bakke, Alan, 129
Baltimore, MD, 124; Mother Rescuers, 139–40
Baltimore Association of Black Caulkers, 40
Baltimore Caulkers Organization, 40
Baptist, Edward, 22
Barber, J. B., 126
Barfield, Clementine, 140
Barnes, Sandra, 148–49
Bechet, Sidney, 147
benefit societies, 40–41, 71, 80, 160. *See also* fraternal orders
Benjamin, Georges C., 154
Bentley-Edwards, Keisha L., 136
Berlin, Ira, 124–25
Berry, Daina Ramey, 14–15
Berry, William, 31
Bethel, Elizabeth Rauh, 70
Bibb, Henry, 23
Biden, Joe, 150
Biggs, Adam, 110
Birmingham, AL: housing segregation in, 62; steel mills, 61
Black AIDS Institute, 145
Black Americans. *See* African Americans
Black and White Men Together (BWMT), 132
Black Coalition Against COVID, 150
"Black Codes," 55
Black Cross Nurses (BCN), 106
Black health care systems: challenges to, 104–5; emergency care, 111–12, *112*; midwifery, 115–17, *116*; National Negro Congress agenda, 106–7; postbellum period, 65–80
Black Lives Matter (BLM) movement, 150, 151
Black Lives Matter Electoral Justice Project, 150
Black nationalist movement, 106
Black Panther ambulance service, 111
Black Panther Party, 111

Black Power movement, 107
Blackwell, Raymond, 100
Black Women in White (Hine), 74
Blakely, Robert L., 14
"blood-type groups," 102
Blue, Carl, 159
Boas, Franz, 78
body-snatching, 15
boll weevils, 56–57
Boston, MA: board of public health, 27; gentrification of, 124; Roxbury community, 144
Braithwaite, Ronald L., 154
Braudel, Fernand, 19
Braun, Lundy, 50
breastfeeding, 9
Brookings Institute, 136
Brooks, Sara, 83
Brotherhood of Sleeping Car Porters, 106
Brown, Eric, 123
Brown, Henry, 21
Brown, John, 12–13
Brown, Leslie, 63, 92–93
Brown Fellowship Society, 40–41
Brown v. Board of Education, 158
Butler, Pierce, 19
Butts, John, 12
Byrd, W. Michael, 25, 38, 47, 76, 87, 127, 128

cadaver trade, 14–15
Cain, William, 22
Calhoun, John C., 37
California Propositions 13 and 209, 121
Callen, Maude, 116
Camp Barker, 48, 69, 72
Campbell, Melanie, 136
Camplin, Moses, 66, 67–68
cancer, 131; mortality rates of, 143–44
Cannon, George D., 102
Cannon, J. Alfred, 126
carceral state. *See* mass incarceration
Carnegie, Andrew, 75
Carnegie Foundation, 78, 79, 80
Carolina or, The Planter (Ogilvie), 19

deindustrialization, 119–20, 123
Delany, Martin R., 35, 37–38, 45
Democratic Party, 142; in Montgomery, AL, 57; in postbellum South, 43, 56
Denton, Nancy, 122
Department of Health and Human Services (DHHS), 126
Depo-Provera (drug), 99
desegregation. *See* segregation
Desmond, Matthew, 123
Detroit, MI: African American mayor of, 142; auto industry, 156–57; deindustrialization of, 120; tuberculosis (TB) rates in, 104
Diallo, Amadou, 125
Diawara, Manthia, 125
Dickerson, Janet, 159
digital age, 119–52; cancer, 131; COVID-19 pandemic, 134–37; grassroots organizing in, 138–40; health care crisis, 143–51; HIV/AIDS epidemic, 131–32; Hurricane Katrina, 132–34; mental health and carceral state, 137–38; modern medical rights movement, 125–30; new service economy, 119–21; sickle cell anemia, 130–31; social justice activism, 140–43; social service systems deterioration, 121–25
dissection of bodies, 11–12
Dix, Dorothea, 10–11
Dixie Hospital Training School, 76
Dodd, Judy, 141–42
Donaldson, John, 66–67
Donelson, A. J., 55
Door, Gregory Michael, 98
Dorchester Home, 71
Douglass, Frederick, 77
Downs, Jim, 44
Drake, Daniel, 26–27
"drapetomania," 3
Drew, Charles, 114
Dublin, Louis I., 85
Du Bois, W. E. B., 153
Duke family, 75

Durham, NC, 63; Lincoln Hospital for Blacks, 75; and tobacco industry, 92
dust inhalation, 18

Ehrenreich, Barbara, 113
Ehrenreich, John, 113
Elders, Joycelyn, 141
Ellis-Hagler, Graylon, 144
emancipation, 43–80; during Civil War period, 43–48, 45, 46; medical segregation, 52–54; postbellum agricultural labor, 55–59; postbellum Black health care system, 65–80; postbellum health care, 48–52; urban industrial health hazards, 59–65
enslavement: background and overview of, 7–8; and communicable disease, 24; and cotton production in Deep South, 21–24; deceased slaves' bodies, 14–15; enslaved persons as capital, 16, 17; enslaved persons as medical healers, 29–32; food production by enslaved persons, 38–39; forced migration, 22; fugitive slaves, 2–3, 44; health in urban industrial contexts, 24–29; hospitalization of enslaved persons, 27–28; illness, 23–24; medicalization of Blackness, 8–11; plantation medical practices, 15–18; plantation production, health consequences of, 18–21; slave labor management policies, 41; statistics of, 42; and unethical experimentation, 11–15, 33–35, 34, 95–99; in urban industrialized contexts, 39–40; and violence against women, 21–25; and whipping, 22–23
environmentalist perspectives of disease, 101–2
environmental racism, 142
epidemics, 25–26; Black service to white population, 41; COVID-19, 134–37; HIV/AIDS, 131–32; influenza (1918–19), 84; smallpox, 53; tuberculosis (TB), 53. *See also* communicable disease

McBride, David, 44, 51, 64, 70, 78, 87–88, 101, 105, 132

McCarty, Margaret "Peggy," 139–40

McDowell, Ephraim, 33

meatpacking industry, 90

Medicaid, 110, 128

Medical and Surgical Observer (journal), 77

Medical Committee for Human Rights (MCHR), 109

medical field, 76; academic health centers (AHCs), 113; African American access to health care, 53–54; African American access to training, 35–38, 88–89; and Black bodies, 14–15; Black enrollment in medical schools, 128; doctor/patient ratios, 104–5; inequities in, 112–14; modern medical rights movement, 125–30; "moral interpretations" of disease, 50; politics and medical rights movement, 107–12; professionalization of, 78–79; professionalization vs. "folk" medicine, 115–17; "quackery," 78; racism in, 50–52. *See also* American Medical Association (AMA)

medical systems, African American, 29–42; Flexner Report on, 79–80; struggle to establish facilities for, 38–42; Western medical training, access to, 35–38; women healers, 32–35

Medicare, 110, 128

Medicine and Slavery (Savitt), 22

Medico-Chirurgical Society of the District of Columbia, 77

Meharry Medical College, 73, 76, 78, 80, 104, 141

Mellon Institute, 101

Memphis, TN: housing crisis in, 103; public health centers in, 87; race riots in, 57

mental illness, 157; and carceral state, 137–38; "Colored Buildings" in asylums, 49–50; definitions of, 2–3; in newly emancipated persons, 48–49;

racial inequities in treatment of, 102; racially biased cures for, 9–10

Mercy Hospital and School for Nurses, 86

Merrick, John, 75

Metropolitan Life Insurance Company, 85

Miami, FL, 62

Middle Passage, 7

midwifery, 32–35, 115–17, 116, 149

migration: from South, 63–64; Black return to urban South, 124–25; forced, 1–2, 22; international immigration to United States, 125; from suburbs, 124. *See also* Great Migration

Milledgeville, GA, 49; Milledgeville State Hospital, 137

Miller, Herbert, 78

minimum wage, 120–21

Minor, John, 21

Minor's Moralist Society, 41

Mississippi State Hospital, 28

Mississippi Summer Project, 109

Mitchell, Roger A., 151

Modern Black Freedom Movement, 104, 107, 110, 119, 121, 123

Modern Black Freedom Struggle, 110, 129–30

Modern Black Liberation Movement, 107

Modern Black Medical Rights Movement, 104–5

Montgomery, AL, 56; forced sterilization court case in, 98–99; retrenchment of by Democrats, 57

Montgomery Community Action Council (MCAC), 98–99

Montgomery Daily Ledger (newspaper), 48

Moore, Aaron M., 75

Moore, Susan, 136

Morais, Herbert M., 47

"moral interpretations" of disease, 50

Morehouse School of Medicine, 140

Morgan, Philip D., 19

Morial, Marc, 134

Morrison, Toni, 147

Mossell, Nathan Francis, 75

Mother Rescuers, 139–40
Mothers of East Los Angeles (MELA), 140
Mothers ROC (Reclaiming Our Children), 140
Mumford, Kevin, 132
Munoz, Cecilia, 135
Murray, Frederick, 141
Murrell, Thomas W., 51, 52
mutual benefit organizations, 40–41, 71. *See also* fraternal orders
Myrdal, Gunnar, 56, 154

NAACP, 105, 109; National Medical Committee, 107
Nagin, Ray, 147–48
Nashville, TN: lynchings in, 58; Meharry Medical College, 73, 76, 78, 80, 104, 141
National Association of Colored Graduate Nurses, 76
National Black Leadership Commission on AIDS (NBLCA), 145
National Black Women's Health Project, 99
National Cancer Institute (NCI), 141
National Center for Health Statistics, 150
National Coalition on Black Civic Participation, 136
National Committee for Mental Hygiene (NCMH), 103
National Domestic Worker's Alliance, 151
national health insurance, 107, 142
National Institutes of Health (NIH), 141
National Medical Association (NMA), 76–77, 107, 127–28; Medical Committee for Civil Rights, 109
National Negro Congress (NNC), 106–7
National Negro Health News (periodical), 105
National Urban League (NUL), 109, 115, 134, 141
Native Americans, 150; and mental illness, 9–10, 11
needle exchange programs, 144

Negro Business League, 105
Negro Health Week, 105–6
Negro's Struggle for Survival, The (Holmes), 102, 114
Negro Year Book (Tuskegee Institute), 58
Nelson, Alondra, 81, 161
New African Free School, 35
New Deal social welfare programs, 88–89
New England Hospital for Women and Children, 73
"New Negro" movement, 105
New Orleans, LA: African American mayor of, 142; African cultural influences in, 147; Common Ground clinic, 145; flooding in (1927), 146; housing stock in, 63; and Hurricane Katrina, 132–34; Phillis Wheatley Club, 71; post-Katrina, 145–46; race riots in, 57; yellow fever epidemics in, 26
New Orleans Medical News and Hospital Gazette, 12
New York City, NY: African American mayor of, 142; gentrification in Harlem, 124; Harlem Hospital, 110; health clinics for activists in, 109; race riots in, 57; tuberculosis (TB) epidemic in, 102; yellow fever epidemics in, 26
New York Manumission Society, 35
New York Urban League, 134
Nichols, Christopher, 23
Norfolk, VA, 28, 71; Black migration to, 83; Mar-Hof textile company, 92; public health center, 86–87
North, Richard L., 9
Nuremberg Code (1947), 98
nurse training school movement, 72–76

Oakland, CA, 123
Obama, Barack, 135, 151
Obamacare, 150–51
O'Donnell Heights Housing project, 140
Office of Economic Opportunity (OEO), 110

Ogier, Thomas L., 68
Ogilvie, George, 19
Ohio Medical Journal, 84
Old North State Medical Society of North Carolina, 77
Overton, Spencer, 150

Paycheck Protection Program (PPP), 137
Peck, David John, 35, 37
pellagra, 64–65
penicillin, 96–97
Pennington, James W. C., 16
Pennsylvania Gazette (newspaper), 30
People's Coalition Against Lead Poisoning, 111
People's Free Medical Centers (PFMCs), 111
Pernick, Martin, 97
Perry, Ivory, 110–11
Personal Responsibility and Work Opportunity Reconciliation Act (1996), 121
Philadelphia, PA: African American mayor of, 142; Black and White Men Together (BWMT), 132; Frederick Douglass Memorial Hospital, 73, 75; Gas Works protest, 140; gentrification of, 124; Henry Phipps Institute, 85; Mercy Hospital and School for Nurses, 86; Phipps Institute medical program, 87; tenement house disaster, 99–100; yellow fever epidemic (1793) in, 26, 41
Philadelphia Negro, The (Du Bois), 153
Philadelphia Record (newspaper), 100
Philadelphia Tribune (newspaper), 100
Phillis Wheatley Club, 71
Phipps Institute, Philadelphia, 87
Pickens, Israel, 21
Pittsburgh, PA: Freedom House Ambulance Service, 111–12, 112; Presbyterian University Hospital, 138, 139; University of Pittsburgh, 141–42; University of Pittsburgh Medical Center (UPMC), 158; Urban League of

Pittsburgh (ULP), 141–42; Wage Review Committee, 159–60
Pittsburgh Courier (newspaper), 106
plantation system, 7; health consequences of, 18–21; medical practices of, 15–18
politics and medical rights movement. *See* medical field
Pond, Cara Scott, 74
Poor Saints Fund, 40
Portsmouth, VA, 71
poverty: concentrated urban, 121, 122; demonization of, 27; racism and "culture of poverty," 98; in Southern states, 57
Price of Their Pound of Flesh, The (Berry), 14
Prince Hall Masonic order, 40
prison systems, 61–62. *See also* mass incarceration
Promised Land community, SC, 47, 59, 70
property ownership, 38–40, 50, 59
Propositions 13 and 209 (CA), 121
Provident Hospital and Nurse Training School (Chicago), 73, 74
public health: community-level efforts for, 70–72; and epidemic prevention efforts, 27; and New Deal, 88–89; public health centers, 86–88; public health movement, 77–78
Pullman Company porters, 93
Purvis, Charles, 72

Quillian, Daniel D., 51–52

Raboteau, Albert, 29
"Race Peculiarities of the Prevalence of Syphilis in Negroes" (essay), 51–52
race riots, 57–58
Race Traits and Tendencies of the American Negro (Hoffman), 51
racial inequities: in health care system, 100–101; in health outcomes, 1; in treatment of mental illness, 10–11
racism: Black inferiority myth, 7, 9, 78, 85, 114, 153; in employment, 120–21;

environmental, 142; and interpretations of disease, 113–14; medical, contemporary, 126–28, 154–55; in medical associations, 76–77; in medical profession, 50–52; in medical science, 41–42, 101–2; mob attacks against Black communities, 58; myth of eliminating African Americans, 51, 85; scientific, 51; systemic and structural, 134–35

Rahim, Malik, 133, 145
railroad construction, 60
Raleigh, NC, 76
Randolph, A. Philip, 106
Rawless, T. K., 114
Red Cross, 106
Redeemer segregationism, 43, 57–58
"red light" districts, 64
Regents of the University of California-Davis v. Bakke, 129
Reich, Steven A., 91
Relf, Minnie, 98–99
Relf v. Weinberger, 98
reproductive rights, 99–100
Republican Party, 43, 55–56
Reuter, Edward, 102
Reverby, Susan M., 96
Reyburn, Robert, 48, 72
rice production, 18–19; and wage labor, 59–60
Richland, VA, 138
Richmond, VA, 56, 71–72
rickets, 64
Rinehart and Dennis (construction firm), 95
Riperton, Minnie, 131
Rivers, Eunice, 96
Robbins, Paul A., 136
Roberts, Samuel Kelton, 84, 88
Robinson, E. I., 107
Rock, John Sweat, 35, 38
Rockefeller, John D., 75
Rockefeller Foundation, 80
Roe v. Wade, 99
Roman, Charles V., 77–78

"root shock," 147
Rosenwald, Julius, 75
Rosenwald Fund, 87–88, 104, 105
Rosner, David, 91, 101
Rowh, Mark, 95
Rush, Benjamin, 8, 41
Rush, Bobby, 112
Russell, Ira, 47

Safar, Peter, 111–12
Samson, Abraham, 100
Sanford, Ezell, 1
San Francisco Bay Area, CA: Black Coalition on AIDS, 145; Black migration to, 83; gentrification of, 124
Santomee, Lucas, 35
Satcher, David, 141
Savannah, GA, 27–28; gentrification of, 124; Men's Sunday Club, 71
Savitt, Todd L., 22, 26
Schoen, Johanna, 98
Scott, Melissa J., 136
Seattle, WA, 83
segregation: and concentrated urban poverty, 122; desegregation of hospitals, 110; in health care systems, 2; in hospitals and infirmaries, 28, 53–54, 56, 73; in housing, 62–63; medical, 52–54, 77, 107–14; in mental health facilities, 11; of Union troops during Civil War, 45–47
Segrest, Mab, 10, 49–50, 102
service economy, 119–21
sexual context of slavery, 21–25
sharecropping system, 54, 55, 56, 57, 70
Shecut, John, 9
Sheppard-Towner Bill, 87
Shoemaker Health Center (Cincinnati), 87
Shufeldt, Robert, 51
Sick and Tired of Being Sick and Tired (Smith), 70–71
sickle cell trait and anemia, 9, 26, 65, 130–31, 143
silica exposure, 95

silicosis, 91
Simkins v. Moses H. Cone Memorial Hospital, 110
Simmons, Robert A., 106
Sims, James Marion, 12–13, *13*, 31, 33, *34*
skin color experimentation, 11–12
Skinner, K. Washington, 22
smallpox, 53
Smith, Bessie, 147
Smith, James McCune, 35–37, *36*
Smith, Susan L., 70–71
Snow, Jennifer, 33
social Darwinism, 101–2, 113, 114
socioeconomic stratification: class-biased social policies, 27; in medical system, 125
SOSAD (Save Our Sons and Daughters), 140
"soundness" concept, 16
South Carolina Gazette (newspaper), 16
Southern Christian Leadership Conference (SCLC), 109
Southern Poverty Law Center (SPLC), 99
Spelman, Laura, 75
Spelman College, 75
Spencer, Herbert, 51
spirometry, 50
Springfield, IL, 57
Spurgeon Jake Winters Free People's Health Clinic, *112*
St. Agnes Hospital, 76
Star in the East Association, 40
Starr, Paul, 50, 54
St. Augustine College for Negroes, 76
steelworkers, 61, 90–91
sterilization, forced, 98–99; and eugenics movement, 103
St. Louis, MO: Homer G. Phillips Hospital, 87, 128; lead poisoning, 111
suburbs, 124. *See also* migration
sugar production, 19–21
Sullivan, Louis W., 140
sunset laws, 56
"Superstition and Health" (survey), 115

surgery and experimentation on enslaved persons, 11–15, 33–35, *34*
syphilis, 51–52; Tuskegee Syphilis Study, 95–98

Tabb, Linda, 159–60
Taylor, Danille, 147–48
Taylor, Dorceta E., 25–26
Taylor, Keeanga-Yamahtta, 123
Taylor, Sandra E., 154
Taylor, Susie King, 44
Tennessee Colored Medical Association, 77
tetanus (lockjaw), 9
textile industry, 120
Thomas, Richard Walter, 89
Thomas, Wilbur, 111
Tidyman, Phillip, 8–9
Till, Emmett, 149
tobacco production, 18, 92–93; and wage labor, 59
Tobey, James A., 84
Toxic Wastes and Race in the United States (report), 142
Treadwell, Henrie M., 154
Trotter, Otis, 83
Trotter, Thelma, 83
Trump, Donald, 151
Truth, Sojourner, 35, 44
tuberculosis (TB), 53, 64, 83, 102; and overcrowded living conditions, 103–4; and public health efforts, 71–72
Tubman, Harriet, 35, 44
Tuckson, Reed, 150
Tuskegee, AL 59
Tuskegee Institute, 73; *Negro Year Book*, 58; Tuskegee Syphilis Study, 95–98, 157

Union Carbide Corporation, 95
United Church of Christ Commission for Racial Justice, 142
Universal Negro Improvement Association (UNIA), 106
University of Pittsburgh Medical Center (UPMC), 158

urban industrialization: and enslaved persons' health, 24–29; health hazards of, 59–65

Urban League, 105–6; Urban League of Pittsburgh (ULP), 141–42

US Census: 1870, mistakes in, 153–54; miscounting of free Blacks, 37

US Communist Party, 106

US. Public Health Service (USPHS), 96–98, 105

vaccines, COVID, 136

vaginal surgery, 12

vagrancy laws, 55

venereal disease, 102, 104. *See also* syphilis

"vice" districts, 64

Villarosa, Linda, 127

violence against women: in enslavement, 21; forced sterilization, 98–99

Vonderlehr, Raymond V., 97

wage labor, 54; and rice production, 59–60; and tobacco production, 59

Wagner-Murray-Dingell bill, 107

Wailoo, Keith, 130–31, 144

Walker, John, 31

War on Poverty, 110

Washington, Booker T., 77, 105

Washington, DC: alley dwellings, 63; Freedmen's Hospital, 72; gentrification of, 124; hospitals, segregation in, 54

Washington, Harriet A., 12, 33

Weightman, Philip, 90

welfare programs, 121

Wells, Ida B., 28

whipping: of enslaved people, 22–23; of free Black workforce, 55

White, Deborah Gray, 23

white allies. *See* interracial alliances

white supremacy: disease/sickness, frameworks of, 7–8; in medical science, 2, 50–51, 101–5

Williams, Daniel Hale, 74, 75, 77–78

Williams, Fannie Barrier, 74

Williams, Jumaane, 134

Williams, Robin M., 154

Wilmington, NC, 57

Wilson, S. David, 100

Wilson, William J., 121, 122

Winant, Gabriel, 158, 159, 160

Wisconsin, 121

Wolfinger, James, 100

women: Black women healers, 32–35; and factory labor, 92; forced sterilization of, 98–99; midwifery, 32–35, 115–17, 116, 149; violence against enslaved, 21

work: in digital age, 119–21; emancipation, 59–62; enslavement, 18–28; in industrial era, 89–95

Work, Monroe N., 71, 78

Wright, Gwendolyn, 137

Wright, Louis, 113–14

yellow fever, 7, 25–26; epidemics, 41

Zimmerman, George, 151